Kathleen Kendall-Tackett, PhD, IBCLC, FAPA

A Breastfeeding-Friendly Approach to Postpartum Depression

A Resource Guide for Health Care Providers

All royalties from the sale of the book go to New Hampshire Breastfeeding Task Force.

Praeclarus Press, LLC

www.PraeclarusPress.com

Praeclarus Press, LLC
2504 Sweetgum Lane
Amarillo, Texas 79124 USA
806-367-9950
www.PraeclarusPress.com

DISCLAIMER
The information contained in this publication is advisory only and is not
intended to replace sound clinical judgment or individualized patient
care. The author disclaims all warranties, whether expressed or implied,
including any warranty as the quality, accuracy, safety, or suitability of
this information for any particular purpose.

ISBN: 978-1-939807-29-8

Cover Design: Ken Tackett
Acquisition & Development: Kathleen Kendall-Tackett
Copy Editing: Chris Tackett
Layout & Design: Nelly Murariu
Operations: Scott Sherwood

TABLE OF CONTENTS

CHAPTER 5

CHAPTER 6

CHAPTER 7

APPENDIX A

APPENDIX B

APPENDIX C

REFERENCES

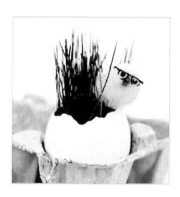

Preface

I wrote the first edition of this resource guide as a curriculum in 2006 after attending a rather dreadful perinatal mental health conference. I was stunned by the way breastfeeding was discussed at this meeting. A presenter from a major east-coast hospital presented for two hours on their comprehensive treatment program for postpartum depression and never mentioned breastfeeding. A practitioner from the Midwest excitedly told me about an OB in her community who was sending all women "at risk" for depression home with an estrogen patch. I tried not to show the horror that I felt and said I thought it was great that this OB was trying to be proactive about postpartum depression. But I expressed my concern that this approach, which is generally not effective when tested in double-blind trails, and was also known to have a deleterious effect on breastfeeding. The tone of the conversation immediately changed, and this practitioner said, "Oh yeah. I forgot. You're the 'breastfeeding one.'" Later that day, another participant said, "YOU speak for the baby. But WE speak for the mother." Wow. So, by supporting breastfeeding, we are only advocating for the baby? That was news to me.

The final comment came following my presentation. An influential practitioner stood and asked me, "don't we need to give mothers permission to wean"? I pointed out that yes, in some cases, that is the best approach. But then I asked her a question. "Can we first ask the mother what is going on? Maybe it's something we can fix."

I came home from that conference feeling very discouraged. I knew that we had been fighting an uphill battle to get the postpartum depression world to even acknowledge breastfeeding, let alone allow for it. But the attitude seemed so negative. I thought of the many mothers I had worked with over the years who were diagnosed with depression and immediately told to wean. They would tearfully tell me, "this is the only thing that is going well for me."

As I pondered this issue, I decided that I needed to act. And with that, the first edition of this resource guide was born.

Fortunately, the story does not stop there. Since 2006, there has been a shift in perinatal mental health. First, practitioners are much more likely to acknowledge breastfeeding—and even support it. Second, recent research has now shown, in a number of studies, that breastfeeding actually protects maternal mental health and lowers women's risk for depression. If a breastfeeding mother gets depressed, breastfeeding helps her cope and also protects her baby from the harmful effects of her depression. One of our recent studies found that breastfeeding even attenuated the impact of sexual assault on all sleep and mental health indices.

It has been thrilling to see these positive changes occur. I want the momentum to continue by providing current evidence that supports this change in paradigm. My goal is that no new mother is told that breastfeeding is causing her depression or that she must wean in order to recover. The choice to wean should be hers alone and we must recognize that breastfeeding can be an important part of her recovery.

The New Hampshire Breastfeeding Task Force sponsored the first two editions of this resource guide. And all royalties on the sales of this Edition will go to them. I have continued to use the bullet-point format because it is easier to read and understand. I have updated the content to reflect recent findings and have added some links to video clips. These can either be accessed online or via smartphones with barcode scanners.

I wish you great success in your work with new mothers. It makes a difference that will last for years.

Kathleen Kendall-Tackett, PhD, IBCLC, FAPA
Amarillo, Texas

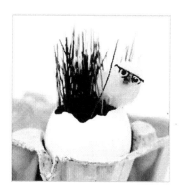

Objectives

After completing this resource guide, you will be able to:

- Identify women who may be at risk for depression in the perinatal period.

- Recognize the important role of breastfeeding in protecting women's mental health and in helping them recover from depression.

- Recognize the symptoms of depression and other mood disorders in pregnant and postpartum women.

- Describe how postpartum mood disorders may impact breastfeeding.

- Describe the causes of postpartum depression.

- Provide information to mothers so they can weigh the risks and benefits of various treatment options for depression.

- Work with mothers to preserve the breastfeeding relationship whenever possible.

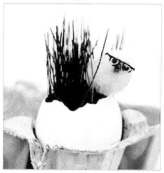

Chapter 1

Towards a Breastfeeding-Friendly Approach to Depression in New Mothers

1. Each year, hundreds of thousands of mothers worldwide become depressed after having a baby.

2. Professionals are more aware of depression than they ever have been, and that's been a positive change. Unfortunately, the number of women with depression is also increasing. Previous estimates were 10% to 20%. Current estimates range from 15% to 25% (Centers for Disease Control, 2008). This increase can be partially explained by increased surveillance, meaning that professionals are identifying more cases. It also could be that more mothers are getting depressed.

3. Perinatal depression and anxiety are common and are major causes of morbidity for both mothers and babies.

4. Depression in pregnancy increases the risk for preterm birth (Coussons-Read, Okun, Schmitt, & Giese, 2005; Dayan et al., 2006).

For example, a prospective study of 681 pregnant women from France found more than twice as many mothers had preterm babies (9.7%) compared with non-depressed women (4%) (Dayan et al., 2006). All the mothers in the study were considered low risk for preterm birth.

5.   Prenatal anxiety had a similar effect in a study of 1,820 women in Baltimore (Orr, 2007). Women with higher rates of anxiety were more likely to have preterm babies.

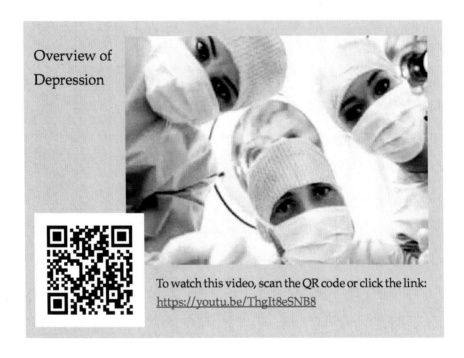

Overview of Depression

To watch this video, scan the QR code or click the link:
https://youtu.be/ThgIt8eSNB8

6.   Maternal depression also has a well-established negative effect on infants and children. Maternal depression is related to problems with children's cognitive, emotional, and social development largely because it influences the way mothers interact with their babies (Kendall-Tackett, 2010b).

7.   The negative effects of maternal depression can last well beyond childhood. A 20-year follow-up study compared adult children of depressed parents to those whose parents were not depressed. The adult children of depressed parents had three times the rate of depression, anxiety disorders, and substance abuse (Weissman, 2006).

8.   The effects of perinatal depression and anxiety are so serious, that several major health organizations have issued policy statements, launched initiatives, and urged practitioners to screen mothers for these disorders. These organizations include:

- The Centers for Disease Control and Prevention, http://www.cdc.gov/reproductivehealth/depression/

- The American Psychological Association, http://www.apa.org/pi/women/programs/depression/ postpartum.aspx

- The American College of Obstetricians and Gynecologists, http://www.acog.org/Patients/FAQs/Postpartum-Depression

- The American Academy of Pediatrics, http://www.aap.org/en-us/about-the-aap/aap-press-room/ Pages/Managing-Maternal-Depression-Before-and-After-Birth.aspx

- The Association of Women's Health, Obstetric, and Neonatal Nurses (AWHONN), http://bit.ly/19xoB89

- The American College of Nurse Midwives, http://www.midwife.org/ACNM/files/ccLibraryFiles/ Filename/000000000659/Postpartum%20Depression.pdf

9. Health care providers are acknowledging the impact of perinatal depression in increasing numbers and are more regularly screening for it. Unfortunately, despite good intentions, some health care providers have attitudes or beliefs about depression that may undermine breastfeeding. Some believe that breastfeeding is expendable—or even the cause of depression. The evidence does not support that position.

10. Recent studies have found that breastfeeding protects maternal mental health and can lower a woman's risk of depression. If a breastfeeding mother gets depressed, breastfeeding can help her recover and establish a positive bond with her baby. For these reasons, it should be preserved whenever possible

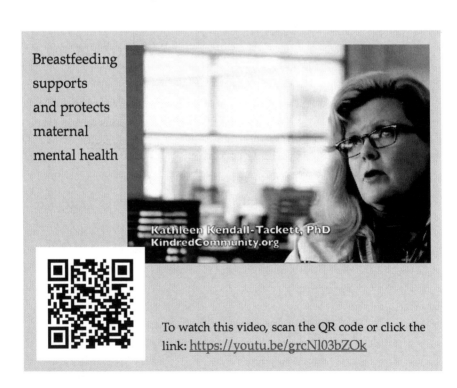

Breastfeeding supports and protects maternal mental health

Kathleen Kendall-Tackett, PhD
KindredCommunity.org

To watch this video, scan the QR code or click the link: https://youtu.be/grcN103bZOk

Chapter 2

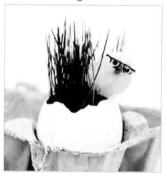

Breastfeeding Protects Mothers and Babies

A. Breastfeeding and Depression

1.   The relationship between breastfeeding and depression is complex. If mothers are depressed during pregnancy or early post-partum, they are more likely to stop breastfeeding. Yet, breastfeeding mothers are at lower risk of depression. Moreover, breastfeeding does not *cause* depression. But breastfeeding problems can.

2.   A qualitative review of 49 articles found that mothers who did not breastfeed were significantly more likely to be depressed (Dennis & McQueen, 2009).

3.   Our study of 6,410 mothers had similar findings. Exclusively breastfeeding mothers had significantly lower depression scores on the Patient Health Questionnaire-2 (PHQ-2) than their mixed- or formula-feeding counterparts. There was no significant difference between mixed- and formula-feeding mothers on any of the measures of depression, sleep, or maternal well-being (Kendall-Tackett, Cong, & Hale, 2011).

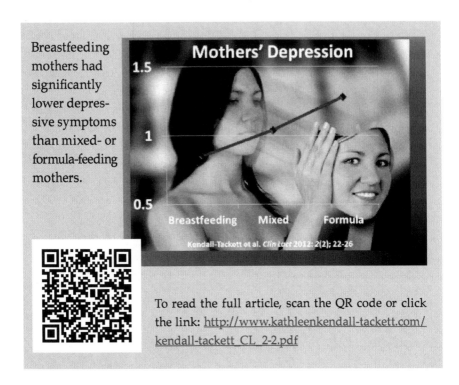

Breastfeeding mothers had significantly lower depressive symptoms than mixed- or formula-feeding mothers.

Mothers' Depression

1.5

1

0.5

Breastfeeding   Mixed   Formula

Kendall-Tackett et al. *Clin Lact* 2012; 2(2); 22-26

To read the full article, scan the QR code or click the link: http://www.kathleenkendall-tackett.com/kendall-tackett_CL_2-2.pdf

4. Breastfeeding *difficulties*, however, may increase the risk of depression. In one study, mothers with nipple pain were significantly more likely to be depressed than women without nipple pain. Once the pain was resolved, mothers were no longer depressed and their moods returned to normal (Amir, Dennerstein, Garland, Fisher, & Farish, 1996).

5. A more recent study with 2,586 mothers found that breastfeeding pain at day 1, week 1, and week 2 were more likely to be depressed at 2 months postpartum (Watkins, Meltzer-Brody, Zolnoun, & Stuebe, 2011). Interestingly, breastfeeding help protects women's mental health when women experienced moderate or severe pain. This study is an example of why breastfeeding support needs to be part of programs to prevent postpartum depression.

6. Breastfeeding may also provide emotional benefits to depressed mothers. Mothers often report that breastfeeding is the "only thing" going well for them, as actress Brooke Shields describes in her story of postpartum depression.

> *If I were to eliminate [breastfeeding], I might have no hope of coming through this nightmare. I was hanging on to breastfeeding as my lifeline.* (Down Came the Rain, p. 80)

Another mother who had postpartum psychosis shared her story with me.

> *What makes me angry is that no one supported me in my desire to breastfeed. I was undermined at every turn by doctors, nurses, even a lactation consultant... It took me three weeks for someone besides my super husband to tell me I was doing a good thing for my baby and a good thing for myself. I was told I just needed sleep, or that I held her too much, or that she wasn't getting enough milk. All I had were people undermining my attempt to breastfeed, all to try and spare me "guilt": "Oh, formula is just fine. It isn't rat poison. Your baby will be happy and healthy, and that's what matters."*
>
> *Well, what about me? What about what I want, and what I want to give my baby? When does what Mom wants come into the picture, rather than what everyone else thinks Mom wants or feels? I have never felt more devalued, more undermined, and less of a person than I did when I had psychosis. Everyone spoke loud and clear, and what they said was, "You can't be a good mom if you breastfeed." You are not a good mom now because you are breastfeeding." Well, they were all wrong. I was sick and I needed help. I needed someone to tell me that, by God, I was a good mom, and that I was doing the best for my baby. I needed someone to offer to do my laundry.*

I needed someone to clean my kitchen, or go to the grocery store. I didn't need any more nonsense about how I would feel better if I just weaned, or if I put the baby on a schedule or any other crap like that (Kendall-Tackett, 2010a).

7. Upon diagnosing depression, health care providers may advise women to wean. For some mothers, that may be the most realistic option. But in most cases, weaning is not necessary. Almost all treatments for depression are compatible with breastfeeding (See Chapter 6). Indeed, some women may refuse to seek treatment because they are afraid that they will be told to wean. Their concern is, unfortunately, realistic (Kendall-Tackett, 2010a).

B. Why Breastfeeding Protects Mothers and Babies

As described in the previous section, breastfeeding protects women's mental health. The next question we may want to ask is why this is so. A key to understanding breastfeeding's protective effect is to understand the human stress response. Breastfeeding protects mothers' mental health because it downregulates—or turns off—the stress response.

1. Stress is a potent risk factor for depression (Kendall-Tackett, 2007). Breastfeeding is adaptive (i.e., confers a survival advantage) because it attenuates, or lessens, the stress response and promotes calm in mothers (Groër et al., 2002; Groër & Morgan, 2007).

2. In a study of 28 mothers who were both breast- and bottle-feeding, researchers measured mothers' mood immediately feeding their babies with either breast or bottle. By studying mothers who were doing both, they accounted for one of the major method-

ological issues in comparing breast- and bottle-feeding mothers (i.e., pre-existing differences between mothers who breast- vs. bottle-feed). Therefore, by having mothers both breast- and bottle-feed in the lab, they were able to determine the impact of feeding type. They found that breastfeeding decreased negative mood, whereas bottle-feeding decreased positive mood, *in the same women* (Mezzacappa & Katkin, 2002).

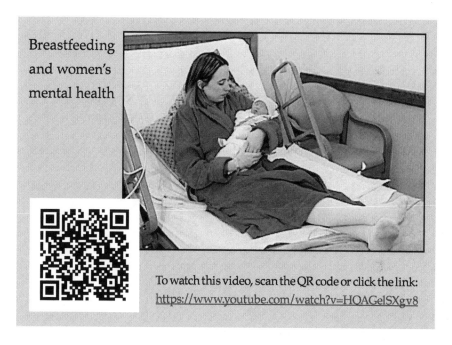

Breastfeeding and women's mental health

To watch this video, scan the QR code or click the link: https://www.youtube.com/watch?v=HQAGelSXgv8

3.   Another study compared the effect of women holding their babies vs. baby at the breast. Holding the babies was good, but baby at the breast led to the biggest reduction in the stress hormones, ACTH and cortisol. In other words, lactation provided a short-term suppression of the HPA axis portion of the stress response (Heinrichs et al., 2001).

4.   Breastfeeding also protects babies' and children's mental health. Maternal depression is stressful for babies because it impacts

the way that mothers interact with their babies (Buss et al., 2012; Grant et al., 2009).

5.   If a mother is depressed, breastfeeding protects her baby. Jones et al. (Jones, McFall, & Diego, 2004) examined the electroencephalogram (EEG) patterns of babies of depressed and non-depressed mothers. (EEG is a way to measure depression in babies.) The EEG patterns of babies of depressed breastfeeding mothers were normal. **In other words, breastfeeding protected the babies of depressed mothers from the harmful effects of maternal depression.**

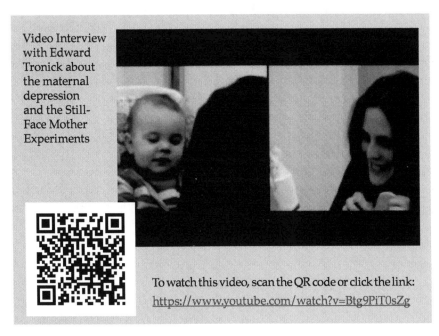

Video Interview with Edward Tronick about the maternal depression and the Still-Face Mother Experiments

To watch this video, scan the QR code or click the link: https://www.youtube.com/watch?v=Btg9PiT0sZg

The authors explained their findings by noting that the depressed/breastfeeding mothers did not disengage from their babies the way that depressed/bottle-feeding mothers did. The depressed/breastfeeding mothers continued to look at, touch, and stroke their babies because these behaviors are built into the breastfeeding relationship.

In contrast, when a mother bottle-feeds, she doesn't have to even hold her baby, making it easier for her to disengage, leading to the symptoms that babies typically exhibit when their mothers are depressed (Jones et al., 2004).

6.   The maternal responsiveness that is necessary in order to breastfeed appears to have a long-term impact on children's mental health. In a 14-year longitudinal study of 2,900 mothers in Western Australia, a dose-response effect of breastfeeding on children's mental health (Oddy et al., 2009). The children were assessed at ages 2, 6, 8, 10, and 14 years. The longer the duration of breastfeeding, the better the child's mental health at every time point. Children's mental was assessed via the Child Behavior Checklist, a measure of child pathology.

7.   Breastfeeding mothers were also significantly less likely to physically abuse or neglect their children than their formula-feeding counterparts (Strathearn, Mamun, Najman, & O'Callaghan, 2009). In a 15-year cohort of 7,223 mother-infant pairs in Australia, there were 512 substantiated cases of maternal-perpetrated child abuse and neglect. Breastfeeding decreased the risk of maternal-perpetrated physical abuse by 2.6 times. Breastfeeding mothers were also 3.8 times less likely to neglect their children.

8.   The authors of this study noted that breastfeeding likely increased oxytocin, with increased mother-infant bonding and lowered mothers' stress and anxiety levels (Strathearn et al., 2009).

9.   This protective effect will be even more protective for mothers with a history of abuse or neglect. In one of our recent studies (Kendall-Tackett, Cong, & Hale, 2013), we had 994 women who reported a history of rape. As predicted, there were pervasive negative effects for all sleep, depression, and well-being measures.

However, when we added feeding method into the equation, we saw that exclusive breastfeeding lessened the effect of sexual assault across each measure. This was not true for mixed- or formula-feeding. We also saw that women with a history of sexual assault breastfed at exactly the same rate as women without a history of sexual assault. (Read the article here. http://www.kathleenkendall-tackett.com/kendall-tackett_bfm_sexual_assault.pdf)

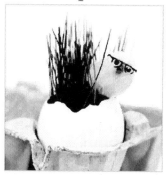

Chapter 3

Consequences of Untreated Postpartum Depression

A. Consequences for Mothers

1. Untreated depression has a profound and devastating impact on the health of mothers and babies. In the most-recent Global Burden of Disease Study, mental disorders, in general, raised the risk of mortality by 2.22 times and shorted life expectancy by an average of 10 years across studies. Depression raised the risk of mortality by 1.71 times (Walker, McGee, & Druss, 2015).

2. Some of the health problems associated with depression are due to the stress hormone cortisol, which is often elevated in people who are depressed. Elevated levels of cortisol can suppress the immune system and lower the number of white blood cells (Kop & Gottdiener, 2005). Increased levels of cortisol can also lead to atrophy of the hippocampus, a brain structure involved in learning and memory. Even formerly depressed patients had smaller hippocampal volume than patients who had never been depressed. The decrease

in volume ranged from 12% to 19% (Sapolsky, 2000).

3.   Elevated cortisol levels can also impact breastfeeding. One study found that high cortisol levels after birth delayed lactogenesis II for several days (Grajeda & Perez-Escamilla, 2002). Lactogenesis II refers to the time when women's milk supply becomes more plentiful three to four days after birth.

4.   Untreated depression also increases the level of systemic inflammation by increasing levels of proinflammatory cytokines (Corwin & Pajer, 2008; Kendall-Tackett, 2007) (see Chapter 4). Increased inflammation is implicated in increased rates of cardiovascular disease, metabolic syndrome, diabetes and other serious chronic diseases in depressed people. For example, patients who become depressed after a myocardial infarction (MI) are three-to-four times more likely to have another MI than those who were not depressed (Lesperance & Frasure-Smith, 2000). Cardiovascular events are less likely in a population of new mothers, but these studies illustrate depression's serious health effects.

5.   Groër and colleagues found that mothers who were stressed, fatigued, or had negative moods had lower levels of prolactin in their milk and serum than mothers who were not tired and stressed. Lower levels of prolactin may have a negative impact on milk supply (Groër et al., 2005; Groër et al., 2005).

6.   Depression also has an impact on women's relationships with their partners. Depressed women are more likely to report poor communication, disengagement, and marital dysfunction that persists long after the depression has resolved (Roux, Anderson, & Roan, 2002).

7.   A study with a community sample of women compared

three groups: those currently depressed, those with a history of depression, and those with no history of depression. The depressed and formerly depressed women were impaired on every measure of interpersonal behavior, had less stable marriages, and lower levels of marital satisfaction than women without a history of depression (Hammen & Brennan, 2002).

B. Consequences for Infants and Children

1. Numerous studies have also demonstrated the harmful effects of maternal depression on infants and children.

2. Mothers with depression or anxiety during pregnancy are more likely to have preterm infants (Dayan et al., 2006; Orr et al., 2008; Wisner et al., 2009).

3. A study of 48 neonates and their mothers (Field et al., 2002) found that infants of depressed mothers had abnormal EEG activation patterns, elevated cortisol levels, and had suboptimum performance on the Brazelton Neonatal Behavior Assessment Scale compared with infants of non-depressed mothers.

4. In a series of two studies, researchers compared infants' cortisol levels after interacting with their depressed or non-depressed mothers (Bugental et al., 2008). The babies were 14 to 16 months old. Infants who had been born prematurely were more reactive to their mothers' depression than were infants who were full-term.

5. In an American sample of 5,000 mother-infant pairs, researchers found that children of depressed mothers had more behavior problems and lower vocabulary scores at age five (Brennan, 2000). In this study, mothers were assessed for depression during pregnancy, immediately postpartum, and at six months and five

years of age. The more severe and chronic the mothers' depression, the more behavior problems the children exhibit.

6. Children of mothers who had postpartum depression were lower in social competence at ages eight to nine in a study from Finland (Luoma, 2001). Social competence included parents' reports of children's activities, hobbies, tasks, and chores; functioning in social relationships; and school achievements. Mothers were assessed for depression prenatally, postnatally, and when their children were eight to nine years old. Mothers' *current* depression was also associated with their children's low social competence and low adaptive functioning.

7. The impact of parental depression can last well past childhood. A 20-year follow-up of children of depressed parents compared them with a matched group of children of parents with no psychiatric illness. The adult children of depressed parents had three times the rate of major depression, anxiety disorders, and substance abuse compared with children of non-depressed parents. In addition, children of depressed parents had higher rates of medical problems and premature mortality (Weissman et al., 2006).

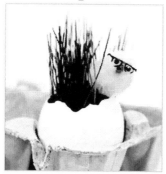

Postpartum Depression and Co-Occurring Conditions

A. Incidence and Symptoms

1.   Perinatal depression is relatively common, affecting approximately 12% to 25% of new mothers worldwide (Beck, 2006; Centers for Disease Control, 2008; Kendall-Tackett, 2010b).

2.   Some populations, however, such as low-income, ethnic-minority mothers, may have rates as high as 40% to 50% (McKee, Cunningham, Jankowski, & Zayas, 2001). However, in cultures that support new mothers, rates of postpartum depression and co-occurring conditions are quite low (Stern & Kruckman, 1983).

3.   Depression may also manifest as somatic complaints or severe fatigue. In many cultures, these symptoms are more acceptable than depression, so depression may present as pain or tiredness. Since sleep is often compromised in the depression, a good screening question to ask is, "How many minutes does it take you to fall asleep?" If it takes longer than 25 minutes, she may be depressed (Kendall-Tackett et al., 2011).

4.   Another indication of possible depression is increased use of health care services for the mother or her baby. If a mother is seeking care above and beyond normal well-care, she may be depressed (Kendall-Tackett, 2010b). Of course, any possible real illness needs to be ruled out before concluding that a mother is simply depressed.

Symptoms of Depression

- Depressed or dysphoric mood

- Anhedonia (inability to experience pleasure in normally pleasurable activities)

- Sleep difficulties unrelated to infant care

- Fatigue

- Inability to concentrate

- Hopelessness

- Changes in appetite

- Increased anger or hostility, and thoughts of death

5.   "Baby blues" are often mild and self-limiting. Many believe, however, that the blues are an early manifestation of depression, and therefore should not be ignored (Beck, 2006).

6.   Postpartum psychosis is relatively rare, occurring in approximately 0.01% of postpartum women. It can manifest as bipolar disorder with psychosis, schizophrenia, or other psychotic states with a postpartum onset. In almost every case, mothers require medications to stabilize their symptoms, and may require hospitalization to ensure their safety and the safety of their babies (Beck, 2006; Kendall-Tackett, 2010b).

B. Co-Occurring Conditions

1. Posttraumatic Stress Disorder (PTSD)

a. Women may experience PTSD or dissociation as a result of a prior trauma-producing event (e.g., childhood abuse, rape or assault, car accident, natural disaster) or as a result of the birth itself (Beck, 2004b).

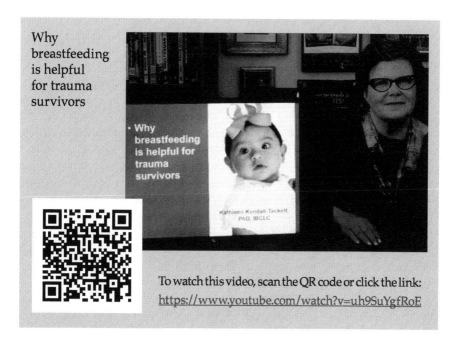

Why breastfeeding is helpful for trauma survivors

To watch this video, scan the QR code or click the link:
https://www.youtube.com/watch?v=uh9SuYgfRoE

b. A key aspect of what makes an event traumatic is whether the mother believed that either she or a loved-one's life was in danger (Beck, 2004a).

c. According to the new diagnostic criteria for PTSD, the person must to be exposed to an event that includes actual or threatened death, actual or threatened injury, actual or threatened sexual violation (Ruglass & Kendall-Tackett, 2015).

d. The event can be directly experienced (the mother), witnessed (partner, doula, nurse, or others), and heard about it happening to a close friend or relative (Ruglass & Kendall-Tackett, 2015).

e. To meet full criteria for PTSD, women must have experienced a traumatic event and have symptoms in four clusters: re-experiencing, avoidance, negative changes in beliefs and mood, and changes in arousal and reactivity (Friedman, Resick, Bryant, & Brewin, 2011; Ruglass & Kendall-Tackett, 2015).

f. Even when someone does not meet full criteria, they may still have symptoms that can be troublesome. For example, emotional numbness or dissociation after a traumatic birth may make it difficult initially for a mother to bond with her baby. Intrusive thoughts, nightmares, and chronic hyperarousal may compromise the quality of a mother's sleep, further impairing her mental health (Beck, 2006; Kendall-Tackett, 2010b).

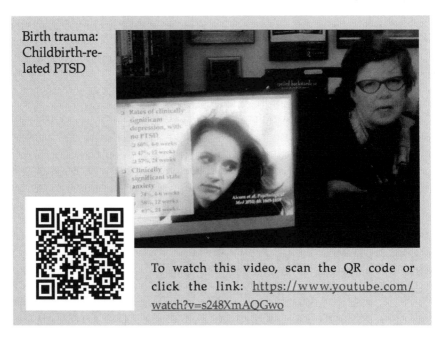

Birth trauma: Childbirth-related PTSD

To watch this video, scan the QR code or click the link: https://www.youtube.com/watch?v=s248XmAQGwo

Risk factors for traumatic childbirth

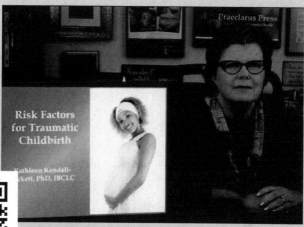

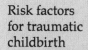

To watch this video, scan the QR code or click the link:
https://www.youtube.com/watch?v=BgcFqVicZwo

Breastfeeding's impact on child abuse and neglect

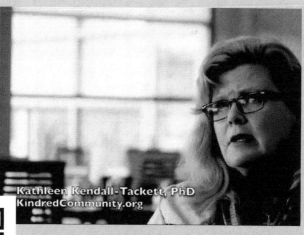

To watch this video, scan the QR code or click the link: https://youtu.be/KgPfqUO4BmY

g. Mothers are more vulnerable to PTSD if they have had prior episodes of depression or PTSD, are abuse survivors (which increases the risk of both PTSD and depression), had prior episodes of loss (including childbearing loss), or were depressed during pregnancy (Ruglass & Kendall-Tackett, 2015).

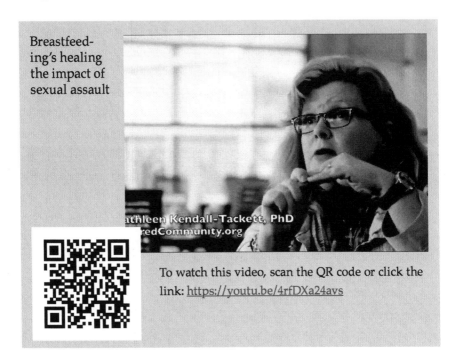

Breastfeeding's healing the impact of sexual assault

To watch this video, scan the QR code or click the link: https://youtu.be/4rfDXa24avs

h. PTSD is more common in ethnic-minority women. In one study of 1,581 pregnant women, African Americans had more lifetime PTSD and trauma exposure, and *almost 4 times the rate of current PTSD* compared to other women in the study (Seng, Kohn-Wood, McPherson, & Sperlich, 2011).

i. African American women were more likely to report symptoms of birth trauma in the Listening to Mothers survey (Declercq, Sakala, Corry, & Applebaum, 2008).

j.   PTSD or depression during pregnancy can also lead to pregnancy complications, including increased rate of miscarriage and premature birth (Seng, Low, Sperlich, Ronis, & Liberzon, 2011). This elevated risk could be related to elevated levels of proinflammatory cytokines, which also ripen the cervix (Coussons-Read et al., 2005; Dayan, 2006).

2. Bipolar Disorder

a.   Bipolar disorder can also manifest in the postpartum period for the first time. The postpartum period is the time of greatest risk for a woman to develop hypomanic symptoms (Yatham et al., 2009).

b.   An underlying postpartum bipolar disorder may be initially misdiagnosed as major depression in the postpartum period. In such situations, if a manic episode is triggered by treatment of depression with an SSRI, a diagnosis of bipolar disorder would likely be more appropriate.

c.   Postpartum bipolar disorder can occur with or without psychosis and tends to run in families. Mothers whose own mothers had bipolar disorder with psychosis are at particularly high risk of experiencing the same condition (Kendall-Tackett, 2010b).

3. Eating Disorders

a.   Eating disorders can occur during pregnancy and the postpartum period.

b.   Active eating disorders during pregnancy or postpartum increase the rate of postpartum depression. In a sample of 49 women with eating disorders who had recently given birth, the rate of postpartum depression was 35% (Franko et al., 2001).

c. Active bulimia nervosa during pregnancy also increased the risk of postpartum depression, miscarriage, and preterm birth (Morgan et al., 2006). The risk of depression (OR 2.8, CI=1,2-2.6), miscarriage (OR=2.6, CI=1.2-5.6), and preterm birth (OR=3.3, CI-1.3-8.8) were all increased among with women with active bulimia. The comparison group was pregnant women with quiescent bulimia.

4. Obsessive-Compulsive Disorder (OCD)

a. OCD is characterized by recurrent, unwelcome thoughts, ideas and doubts and/or the presence of compulsive behaviors. The exact incidence of postpartum OCD is not known, but a high percentage of women with postpartum OCD also have postpartum depression.

b. Postpartum OCD can manifest itself as repetitive thoughts of infant harm or intrusive images of accidental harm to the baby. Unlike women with psychosis, women with postpartum OCD are usually appalled and frightened by their thoughts, and will go to extreme measures to keep something from happening to their infants (Abramowitz et al., 2002).

c. In contrast, women with postpartum psychosis are out of touch with reality, and may experience delusions that external forces are telling them to harm their infants, and thus, are at grave risk of hurting themselves or their children (Beck, 2006). Postpartum psychosis is an acute clinical emergency that requires immediate medical care to assure the safety of both mother and baby.

d. OCD and co-occurring depression are treated with SSRIs.

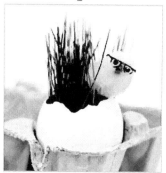

Chapter 5

Causes of Depression in New Mothers

- The factors that underlay depression in mothers vary from woman to woman. Each of these risk factors alone can cause depression. However, many mothers have multiple risk factors and these can potentiate each other.

- Causes of depression in new mothers fall into five categories. These are listed below. By helping mothers identify the sources of their depression, intervention can be targeted more specifically.

A. Physiological Causes

1. Inflammation in Depression

a. Researchers have discovered that systemic inflammation has an important role in the etiology of depression in new mothers and may, in fact, underlie the other known risk factors (Kendall-Tackett, 2007).

b.   Inflammation includes high levels of proinflammatory cyto-kines and acute-phase proteins, such as C-reactive protein (CRP), in the mother's plasma (Kop & Gottdiener, 2005). The cytokines that have been most consistently identified in depression are inter-leukin-1β (IL-1β), interleukin-6 (IL-6), and tumor necrosis factor-α (TNF-α).

c.   Cytokines are the chemical messengers of the white blood cells. In preparation for birth, levels of proinflammatory cytokines rise during the last trimester of pregnancy. When these cytokines are within normal levels, they are adaptive because they help prevent infection, and prepare women's bodies for labor. When they are abnormally high, however, they increase the risk of depression and a number of serious illnesses (Kiecolt-Glaser et al., 2007; Maes, Bosmans, & Ombelet, 2004; Robles, Glaser, & Kiecolt-Glaser, 2005).

d.   There are a number of reasons why inflammation increases the risk of depression. First, when inflammation levels are high, people experience classic symptoms of depression, such as fatigue, lethargy, and social withdrawal.

e.   Second, inflammation increases levels of cortisol—a stress hormone that is often elevated in depressed people. And finally, inflammation decreases the neurotransmitter serotonin by lowering levels of its precursor, tryptophan (Corwin, Bozoky, Pugh, & John-ston, 2003; Maes, & Smith, 1998).

f.   To read more about inflammation and postpartum depres-sion, click here, http://www.internationalbreastfeedingjournal.com/content/2/1/6

2. Fatigue/Sleep Disturbance

a. Fatigue and sleep difficulties can both cause and be a consequence of depression.

b. Depression alters and impairs sleep (Posmontier, 2008). Depressed mothers get less sleep and poorer-quality sleep than their non-depressed counterparts, even when the baby is not with them (Field et al., 2007; Lee, Lee, Rankin, Weiss, & Alkon, 2007).

c. Separation of mother and baby to prevent or treat depression may not be effective because depressed mothers' sleep is likely to be disturbed, even if their babies are not there.

d. Exclusively breastfeeding mothers get more sleep and report less daytime fatigue and lower rates of depression in a sample 6,410 new mothers (Kendall-Tackett et al., 2011). Below are our findings.

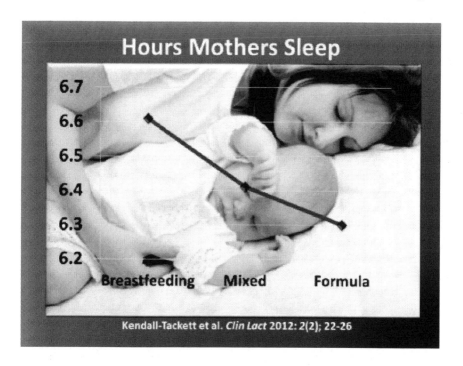

Hours Mothers Sleep

Kendall-Tackett et al. *Clin Lact* 2012: 2(2); 22-26

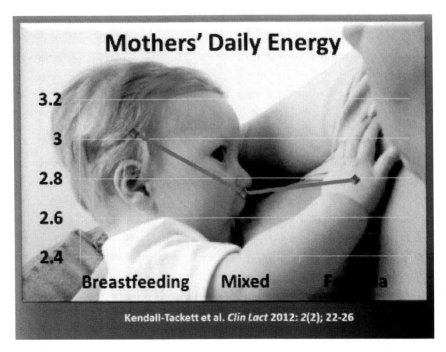

e. In the Kendall-Tackett et al. study, there was no significant difference, on any variable, between the mixed- and formula-feeding mothers (Kendall-Tackett et al., 2011). This suggests that mothers who supplement will likely get less rest and be more tired. Supplementation is not a good long-term strategy for mothers who are extremely fatigued. [Read the full article here, http://www. kathleenkendall-tackett.com/kendall-tackett_CL_2-2.pdf

f. Inflammation is related to fatigue and depression. When inflammation is high, mothers become fatigued. And when fatigue is high, inflammation increases. One study found that higher levels of IL-1β were related to fatigue in women at four weeks postpartum (Corwin et al., 2003).

g. The number of minutes that it takes mothers to fall asleep is an important indicator of her mental and emotional health. If it takes a mother 25 minutes to fall asleep, she is at high risk for depression (Goyal, Gay, & Lee, 2007; Kendall-Tackett et al., 2011). **Asking mothers how many minutes it takes to fall asleep is a good, non-intrusive way to assess their emotional state.**

h. Mothers taking medications to help them sleep should never bedshare with their babies.

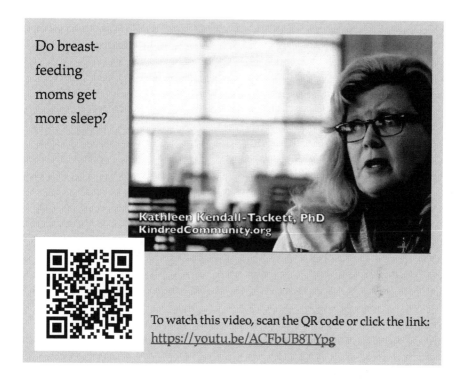

Do breast-feeding moms get more sleep?

Kathleen Kendall-Tackett, PhD
KindredCommunity.org

To watch this video, scan the QR code or click the link:
https://youtu.be/ACFbUB8TYpg

3. Pain

a. Pain and depression are highly co-morbid conditions and may have a common etiology (Kendall-Tackett, 2013).

b. There are many types of pain that postpartum women can experience. Pain can be the result of birth or breastfeeding difficulties. It can be caused by prior psychological trauma, which can lower the pain threshold so that normal sensations are perceived as painful (Kendall-Tackett, 2013).

c. Pain may also trigger depression. High levels of acute pain immediately postpartum tripled the risk of postpartum depression at 3 months for all types of births in another study of 1,288 women (Eisenach et al., 2008).

d. A study of 113 breastfeeding women (48 with nipple pain, 65 without) demonstrated that women with nipple pain were significantly more likely to be depressed than women without pain (38% vs. 14%). Once the pain resolved, their moods returned to normal (Amir et al., 1996). A more recent study of 2,568 women in the U.S. found that breastfeeding pain that early breastfeeding pain (day 1, week 1, week 2) was related to increased risk of postpartum depression at 2 months (Watkins et al., 2011). But breastfeeding help protected mothers' mental health, even when the mothers had moderate-to-severe pain.

e. High levels of proinflammatory cytokines increase pain. Cytokines (especially IL-1) are stimulated by Substance P. Substance P is the neuropeptide present in patients with pain. High levels of Substance P are related to lower levels of serotonin, which increases the risk of depression. Cytokines also increase prostaglandin synthesis, including the prostaglandin cyclooxygenase-2 (COX-2), which increases pain (Konsman, 2002).

4. Reproductive Hormones

a. The hormonal explanation for postpartum depression has limited scientific support. Some of this may be due to inaccurate measures of fluctuating hormones. Future studies may find that reproductive hormones are indirectly related to depression because of their influence on stress hormones, immune markers, or sleep quality.

b. Ahokas and colleagues (Ahokas, Aito, & Rimon, 2000; 2001) have used 17β-Estradiol to treat severe postpartum depression. In one study, 23 women with postpartum major depression were recruited from a psychiatric emergency unit. All were severely depressed and had low serum estradiol concentrations. Within a week of treatment with estradiol, the depressive symptoms had substantially diminished. By the end of the second week, when estradiol levels were comparable to the follicular phase, the scores on the depression measure were comparable to clinical recovery (Ahokas et al., 2001). However, this was an open-label trial and did not account for the placebo effect, so these findings have limited generalizability. Blinded-placebo trials of estrogen, estradiol, or progesterone generally show no improvement in symptoms compared to the placebo (Kendall-Tackett, 2010b).

c. There is not sufficient evidence to support treatment of postpartum depression with estrogen or its metabolites. Estrogen has a dramatic negative impact on milk supply and can lead to breastfeeding cessation (Hale, 2010). This effect, coupled with the lack of empirical support for its efficacy, are sufficient to recommend avoiding estrogen and estradiol as treatments for depression in new mothers.

B. Birth Trauma and Childbirth-Related PTSD

1. A relatively high percentage of women in the U.S. perceive one or more of their birth experiences negatively. In the recent Listening to Mothers II Survey, which included 1,371 mothers online and 200 phone interviews, 9% met full criteria for PTSD, and 18% scored above the cutoff for posttraumatic stress symptoms (Beck, Gable, Sakala, & Declercq, 2011).

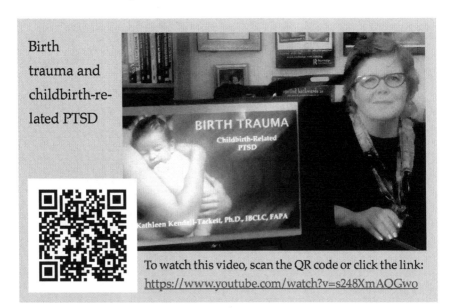

Birth trauma and childbirth-related PTSD

To watch this video, scan the QR code or click the link:
https://www.youtube.com/watch?v=s248XmAOGwo

2.   The rate of full-criteria is higher for women experiencing birth trauma than it was for residents of lower Manhattan following 9/11 (Galea et al., 2003). Beck et al. described this number as a "sobering statistic" (Beck et al., 2011).

3.   In contrast, when women give birth in countries where birth is treated as a normal event and they have continuous labor support, their rates of PTSD are substantially less. For example, the rate of PTSD following birth was 1.3% in Sweden (Soderquist, Wijma, Thorbert, & Wijma, 2009) and 1.9% in the Netherlands (Stramrood et al., 2011).

4.   When women give birth in countries where the status of women is generally low, their rates of PTSD following childbirth are high. For example, in a sample of 400 women from Iran, 55% described their births as "traumatic" and 20% met full criteria for PTSD (Modarres, Afrasiabi, Rahnama, & Montazeri, 2012).

5.   Even if mothers do not have PTSD, they may have depression or anxiety. In a prospective study of 933 pregnant women, rates of full-criteria PTSD in this study ranged from 3.6% to 6.3% across the multiple assessment points. Even when they did not have PTSD, they did not avoid complications. In this sample, 47% to 66% had clinically significant depression, and 58% to 74% had clinically significant anxiety (Alcorn, O'Donovan, Patrick, Creedy, & Devilly, 2010).

6.   Objective aspects of birth (e.g., cesarean vs. vaginal) only account for some reactions. Mothers who have cesarean births are at somewhat increased risk of having a negative reaction, but this is not always true. Subjective aspects of birth, such as those that are listed below, are more likely to lead to a woman's negative assessment of her birth (Beck, 2004b; Kendall-Tackett, 2014a).

- Did she feel her birth was dangerous to herself or her baby?

- Did she feel in control of either the medical situation or herself during labor?

- Did she feel supported during labor and birth?

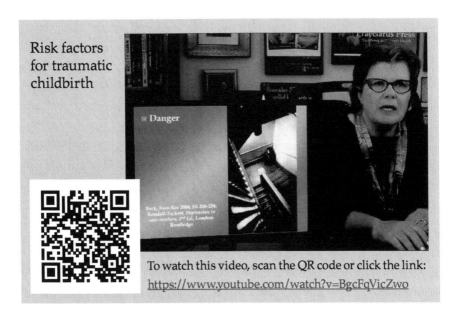

Risk factors for traumatic childbirth

To watch this video, scan the QR code or click the link:
https://www.youtube.com/watch?v=BgcFqVicZwo

7. In a meta-ethnography of 10 qualitative studies, women reported that they often felt traumatized as a result of the actions or inactions of midwives, nurses, and doctors. The care they received was sometimes experienced as dehumanizing, disrespectful, and uncaring (Elmir, Schmied, Wilkes, & Jackson, 2010).

8. Women were more likely to describe their births negatively if they felt "invisible and out of control." They used phrases such as "barbaric," "intrusive," "horrific," "inhumane," and "degrading." Women were also distressed when large numbers of people were invited to watch the birth without their consent (Elmir et al., 2010).

9.   Women felt out of control, powerless, vulnerable, and unable to make informed decisions about their care. They felt betrayed. Some women agreed to procedures, such as epidurals and vacuum extractions, in an attempt to end the trauma they were experiencing (Elmir et al., 2010).

10. In a national survey of 5,332 mothers in the UK, women who had forceps-assisted and unplanned cesareans had the poorest health and well-being overall. Women who had forceps deliveries had the highest rates of symptoms of PTSD, depression, and anxiety. Breastfeeding difficulties were more common in forceps-delivery and unplanned cesareans (Rowlands & Redshaw, 2012).

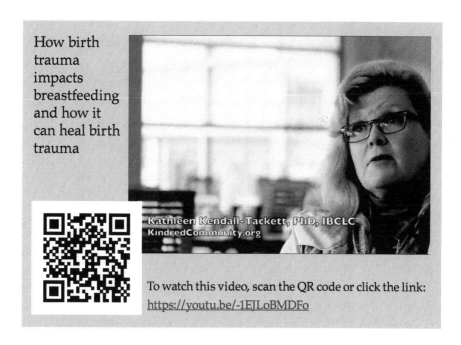

How birth trauma impacts breastfeeding and how it can heal birth trauma

Kathleen Kendall-Tackett, PhD, IBCLC
KindredCommunity.org

To watch this video, scan the QR code or click the link: https://youtu.be/-1EJLoBMDFo

11. Birth trauma can also have an impact on breastfeeding. Beck and Watson (2008), in their qualitative study, found that birth trauma's impact on breastfeeding can lead women down two

strikingly different paths. One can propel women into persevering in breastfeeding. The other can lead to distressing impediments that curtailed women's breastfeeding attempts.

12. In another study, breastfeeding provided an opportunity for some women to overcome the trauma of their birth experiences and "prove" their success as mothers (Elmir et al., 2010), as this mother describes.

> *Breastfeeding became my focus for overcoming the birth and proving to everyone else and mostly to myself that there was something that I could do right. It was part of my crusade, so to speak, to prove myself as a mother* (Beck & Watson, 2008).

13. There are a number of interventions that are effective for treating birth trauma. They include eye-movement desensitization and reprocessing (EMDR), cognitive-behavioral therapy, and expressive writing and journaling, acupuncture, and mindfulness (Kendall-Tackett, 2014b; Ruglass & Kendall-Tackett, 2015).

14. To read more on traumatic childbirth, see the following full-text articles available here, http://www.kathleenkendall-tackett.com/kendall-tackett_birth_trauma.pdf (Kendall-Tackett, 2014a) and here, http://www.kathleenkendall-tackett.com/kendall-tackett_birth_trauma_intervention.pdf (Kendall-Tackett, 2014b).

C. Infant Characteristics

1. Infants with a "difficult" or high-needs temperament increase the risk depression in mothers. These babies are often highly sensitive to their surroundings, don't fall into regular schedules or routines, cry a lot in the first few months, have an intense need to be with their mothers, and often do not sleep well at night.

2.   High-needs babies can undermine a woman's sense of competence and self-efficacy, especially if this is her first baby. In one study, low self-efficacy mediated the effect of temperament on maternal depression. In other words, difficult temperament caused the mothers' depression by making them feel incompetent (Kendall-Tackett, 2010b).

3.   Infant illness, prematurity and disability can also cause depression, acute stress disorder, and PTSD in mothers, particularly if the babies are at high risk. However, this reaction is often delayed, and may not manifest itself until the babies are out of danger. Mothers could become depressed several months after their babies are discharged (Kendall-Tackett, 2010b).

4.   In a study of 21 mothers of very low birthweight infant in Quebec found that 23% were in the clinical range for PTSD when the babies were 6 months corrected age (Feeley et al., 2011). Severity of illness in the infant was related to the mothers' symptoms.

5.   Two effective interventions for mothers of premature infants include assignment of a "buddy," a mother who has also had a preterm infant, and Kangaroo Care (Feldman, Eidelman, Sirota, & Weller, 2002).

6.   A recent randomized, controlled trial compared parent support vs. usual care for mothers of preterm infants. Mothers in the intervention group received crisis intervention at 5 days postpartum. This intervention took place in the NICU, two times a week, for 5 to 15 minutes per session. At discharge, mothers in the intervention group had significantly lower symptoms of depression and anxiety in the intervention mothers (Jotzo & Poets, 2005).

7.   The components of the Jotzo and Poets (2005) intervention included the following elements: reconstruction of events before and

after the birth; provision of relaxation techniques; explanation of stress and trauma; provision of support during "emotional outbursts"; discussion of personal resources and current support; and possible solutions for concrete problems.

D. Psychological Factors

1. Attributional Style

Attributional style refers to how people explain events in their lives. Are they optimists or pessimists? Pessimists attribute negative events to some inherent flaw in themselves, see negative situations as unchangeable, and think that negative events influence every aspect of their lives. These beliefs increase the risk of depression and are specifically addressed in cognitive-behavioral therapy.

2. Previous Psychiatric History

a.   A mother who has had prior episodes of depression or PTSD is at increased risk for depression postpartum (Kendall-Tackett, 2010b).

b.   Researchers have also found that depression in pregnancy is a strong risk factor for postpartum depression (Beck, 2001). In a large sample (N=9,028), depression rates were highest at 32 weeks gestation and lowest at eight months postpartum (Evans, Heron, Francomb, Oke, & Golding, 2001).

c.   Kiecolt-Glaser et al. (2007) noted that a prior history of affective disorders seems to "prime" the inflammatory response, so that the woman's body responds with an exaggerated response when presented with a current stressor. This increased inflammation makes mothers more vulnerable to subsequent stressors, and therefore, more likely to become depressed. However, this elevated risk does not mean depression is inevitable. With proper support for the mother, depression can be avoided.

3. Self-esteem, Self-efficacy, and Expectations

Self-esteem, self-efficacy, and expectations refer to how mothers feel about themselves as mothers. Do they feel competent? Are their expectations for themselves and their babies realistic? Feeling incompetent and having unrealistic expectations both increase the risk of depression.

E. Social Factors

1. Abusive or Dysfunctional Family of Origin

a.   An abusive or dysfunctional family of origin can also increase the risk of depression, as can a history of sexual assault (Kendall-Tackett, 2010b; Kendall-Tackett et al., 2013). Current research includes a broad range of difficulties in mothers' families of origin that can increase the risk of depression, anxiety, substance abuse, or other problems.

b.   These difficulties include child abuse and neglect; parental substance abuse, mental illness or criminal activity; or parental domestic abuse. These types of experiences are referred to collectively as Adverse Childhood Experiences (ACEs). Each of these increases the risk of depression. However, in combination, they are even more harmful.

c.   Adverse Childhood Experiences (ACE) are common. In one sample of more than 17,000 middle-class patients in the U.S., 51% had experienced at least one type of ACE (Felitti et al., 2001). Samples with higher-risk populations tend to have even higher rates.

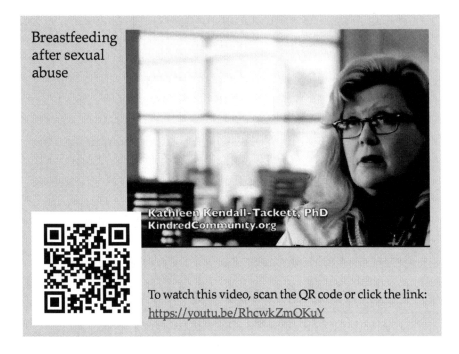

Breastfeeding after sexual abuse

Kathleen Kendall-Tackett, PhD
KindredCommunity.org

To watch this video, scan the QR code or click the link:
https://youtu.be/RhcwkZmOKuY

d. These types of experiences can impact mothers postpartum, most notably by increasing the risk of depression, anxiety, and PTSD.

e. A 25-year longitudinal study of 1,265 adults in Christchurch, New Zealand found an increased risk of depression, anxiety disorders, conduct/anti-social personality disorders, substance abuse, suicidal ideation, and suicide attempts during adolescence among those who experienced childhood physical or sexual abuse (Fergusson, Boden, & Horwood, 2008). Those who had experienced child sexual abuse had 2.4 times higher rates of mental disorders than non-exposed individuals.

f. A study of 6,410 found that 994 had histories of sexual assault (Kendall-Tackett et al., 2013). Sexual assault had a pervasive, negative effect across several domains. The sexually assaulted women had higher rates of depression, more sleep problems (longer to get to sleep, lower overall sleep time, and more night awakenings), more anger and irritability, and more anxiety.

g.   However, when feeding method was added to the analyses, if the sexual-assault survivors were exclusively breastfeeding, the effects of the sexual assault were attenuated. *In other words, exclusive breastfeeding lessened the negative effects of sexual assault for these mothers. These mothers had significantly lower rates of depression, anxiety, anger* and irritability, and significantly better sleep than sexually assaulted women who were mixed- or formula-feeding (Kendall-Tackett et al., 2013).

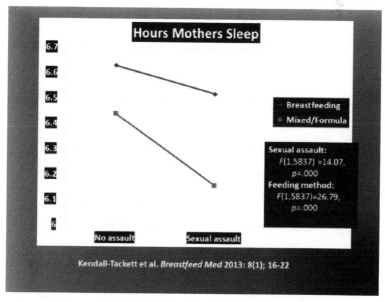

h.   Sexually assaulted women breastfed at exactly the same rates as non-assaulted women: 78% for both groups (Kendall-Tackett et al., 2013). This is consistent with previous studies that have found higher rates of intention to breastfeeding (Benedict, Paine, & Paine, 1994), and breastfeeding initiation (Prentice, Lu, Lange, & Halfon, 2002) for women with a history of child sexual abuse.

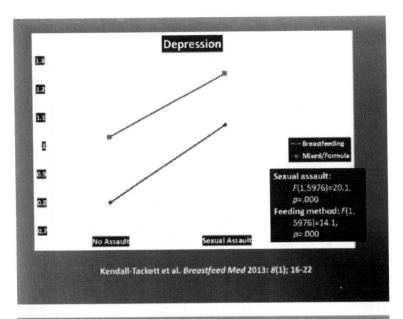

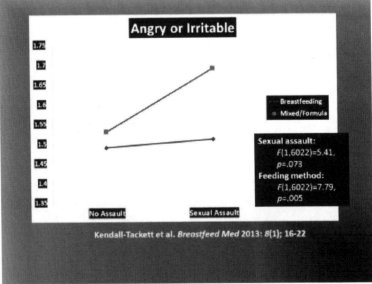

i.   With regard to breastfeeding, it is important not to assume that a mother with a sexual assault history will not want to breastfeed. That will be true for some, but not for others. The women who do choose to breastfeed may still encounter difficulties. Some modifications to breastfeeding, such as limiting skin-to-skin contact, can help women with a history of sexual assault breastfeed. But the most important thing is to find out what the mother wants to do and work from there.

2. Social Support

a. Lack of social support increases the risk of depression. Social support includes emotional and instrumental support, and can be provided by a woman's partner, friends, relatives, and professionals. For women without partner support, support from others can prevent depression (Stern & Kruckman, 1983).

b. Many industrialized cultures lack the supportive and sustaining aspects of community inherent in more traditional non-Western societies (Stern & Kruckman, 1983). But individual practitioners can help new mothers seek this type of support for themselves by offering referrals to mothering organizations and support groups, providing mothers with a realistic picture of what they can expect postpartum, and giving them "permission" to ask for help.

c. Social support is one of the critical factors that increases breastfeeding rates (U.S. Department of Health and Human Services, 2011). Providing it will also lower the risk of depression.

3. Socioeconomic Status

Socioeconomic status can also impact depression. Despite the popular myth, postpartum depression is not more common in White, middle-class women. Lower-income women are more vulnerable to depression (unless they have good support). And when low-income women become depressed, they often have fewer resources available to help them recover (Kendall-Tackett, 2010b).

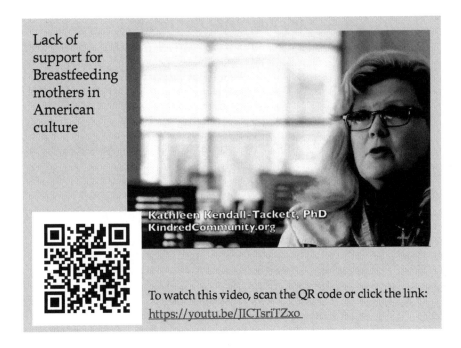

Lack of support for Breastfeeding mothers in American culture

Kathleen Kendall-Tackett, PhD
KindredCommunity.org

To watch this video, scan the QR code or click the link: https://youtu.be/JICTsriTZxo

4. Stressful Life Events

a. Stressful life events refers to the number of life changes a mother has experienced in the past year or so. Having a baby is a significant life stress, and even if perceived positively, may increase the risk of depression because of the magnitude of life changes involved.

b. Mothers who have endured additional recent stressful events, even positive ones (e.g., moving to a new home), are at increased risk of depression.

c. One specific type of life stress is acculturation. Acculturation refers to the cultural adaptation people experience when they immigrate to a new country, often due to fleeing a war or other political situations that makes life in their home country untenable.

Some aspects of acculturation include ability to perform adequate skills for the new country while preserving their own culture, socially integrating into their new society, and having a sense of loss concerning their country of origin (Knipscheer & Kleber, 2006).

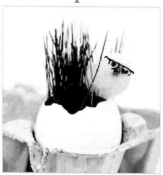

Chapter 6

Assessment of Postpartum Depression

A. Screening for Postpartum Depression

Since pregnancy and postpartum are critical periods of vulnerability, they are also good times for practitioners to screen for depression.Pediatric and obstetric practitioners, nurses, lactation specialists, and peer counselors can all screen for depression.

Screening can be done in prenatal, hospital, home, and pediatric settings. Observation alone is not enough to screen for depression, as many cases will be missed.

Using a standardized scale, such as those described in Section B, results in higher rates of detection.

1. Prenatal Settings

Screening for depression with a risk-assessment tool at the first prenatal visit provides an opportunity to discuss the signs and symptoms of depression in pregnancy and postpartum as mothers enter the health care system. By increasing awareness about perinatal emotional reactions, mothers and their providers can anticipate and proactively address potential issues before they develop. Also, this discussion can help to normalize and decrease stigma about acknowledging emotional difficulties.

2. Hospital Settings

Completing a depression assessment just before discharge from the hospital is a reliable method of identifying possible depression in the immediate postpartum period.

Health care providers should look for subtle signs of depression and offer appropriate referrals. Early screening can help minimize it and the necessity of long-term treatment. Indeed, universal screening may soon become mandatory in health care settings in the U.S. and other countries.

Supporting and teaching mothers the necessity of rest, and finding good social support, may also minimize risk or prevent the escalation of depression.

Red-Flag Symptoms

The mother:

- Has not slept in two or three days
- Is losing weight rapidly
- Cannot get out of bed
- Is ignoring basic grooming
- Seems hopeless
- Says her children would be better off without her
- Is actively abusing substances
- Makes strange or bizarre statements (e.g., plans to give her children away to strangers)

Edinburgh Postnatal Depression Scale-Three-Item Version (EPDS-3)

In the past 7 days,

I have blamed myself unnecessarily when things went wrong
- Yes, most of the time (3)
- Yes, some of the time (2)
- Not very often (1)
- No, never (0)

I have been anxious or worried for no good reason
- Yes, quite a lot (3)
- Yes, sometimes (2)
- No, not much (1)
- No, not at all (0)

I have felt scared and panicky for no very good reason
- No, not at all (0)
- Hardly ever (1)
- Yes, sometimes (2)
- Yes, very often (3)

Scores >3 warrant further screening

(Kabir, Sheeder, & Kelly, 2008)

3. Home Health Setting

Home health nurses or home visitors can be alert for early signs of depression, screen for it, and make referrals as appropriate.

4. Pediatric Office Visits

Heneghan and colleagues (2007) noted that pediatricians see infants approximately seven times in the first year for well-baby checks, making it quite feasible for pediatric providers to identify maternal depression.

The three most common scales to screen for postpartum depression are the PHQ-2, Edinburgh Postnatal Depression Scale (EPDS) and (Cheryl) Beck's Postpartum Depression Screening Scale (PDSS). According to a recent review, both were accurate in identifying depression with a low false-positive rate. These instruments were also more sensitive than instruments that screened for depression in general, such as the (Aaron) Beck Depression Inventory (Gaynes et al., 2005). A recent study found that three items from the EPDS (see above) were more accurate than the full 10-item scale (Kabir et al., 2008).

B. Assessment Inventories

1. Patient-Health Questionnaire-2 (PHQ-2)

a. The 2-item Patient Health Questionnaire (PHQ-2) is a reliable initial health screening that can be used in all health care settings.

Patient Health Questionnaire-2 (PHQ-2)

Over the past two weeks, how often have you been bothered by any of the following problems?

• Little interest or pleasure in doing things
• Feeling down, depressed or hopeless

The response categories include *Not at All (0)*, *Several Days (1)*, *More than Half the Days (2)*, and *Nearly Every Day (3)* and are scored from 0 to 3. The higher the number, the higher the risk of depression.

The PHQ-2 includes the following two questions, and assesses frequency of anhedonia (little interest or pleasure in doing things) and depressed mood (feeling down, depressed or hopeless) during the past two weeks.

b. The PHQ-2 is designed to screen for depression in general, and can be used as a quick screen. A recent study found that it was highly sensitive for identifying postpartum depression during well-child visits (Gjerdingen, Crow, McGovern, Miner, & Center, 2009).

2. Edinburgh Postnatal Depression Scale (EPDS)

The EPDS is the most commonly used postpartum depression screening tool in the world. A complete copy is in Appendix B. The EPDS is a 10-item self-report questionnaire that can be completed in five minutes (Cox, Holden, & Sagovsky, 1987). It was designed to give primary care providers, and other health care workers, a simple tool for screening in the postpartum period.

Women are asked to report how they have felt in the past week, and the items are scored from 0 to 3. A score greater than 12 indicates possible depression (although, some recommend a cutoff of 9 for screening). See Appendix B.

The EPDS offers a number of advantages. It is easy to complete and score, and is specifically written for new mothers. Although, widely used, however, it is written in British rather than American English. American mothers, especially those with lower literacy levels, may find the wording of some of the questions confusing or a little odd.

3. Postpartum Depression Screening Scale (PDSS)

Another screening tool, which offers more depth, is the Postpartum Depression Screening Scale. The PDSS is a 35-item scale. Mothers answer questions about how they feel after birth with their answers ranging from "strongly agree" to "strongly disagree" (Beck & Gable, 2000). It is available at Western Psychological Services. This is a more comprehensive scale that can be used both in clinical practice and research studies. It is also written in American English, so mothers in North America may find it easier to use.

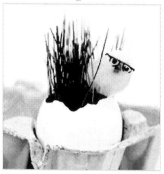

Chapter 7

Treatment Options

A. Creating a Breastfeeding-Friendly Treatment Plan

- There are a variety of effective treatments available for mild, moderate, and severe depression. Breastfeeding-friendly treatment for depression includes a range of conventional and alternative treatments. These can be combined or used separately.

- A breastfeeding-friendly approach to treatment of depression also empowers mothers to weigh their options and make the best treatment choices for themselves and their babies. To achieve that goal, mothers need to be involved in all parts of the decision-making process when it comes to their care. Before suggesting any treatment, talk with mothers about the treatment modalities they are most comfortable with. If mothers feel that their concerns and wishes are not taken seriously, they are less likely to comply with treatment.

- Some mothers are adamant about not using antidepressants and will not take them, no matter what their health care providers say. In the general population of patients with depression, non-compliance rates with antidepressant use are high. In one study of antidepressant use, by the 3-month follow up, only 28% were still taking their medications (Olfson, Marcus, Tedeschi, & Wan, 2006).

- While some mothers may never take medications while breast- feeding, others will if they are assured that the medications will not harm their babies. In this case, patient education is critical. One thing you can do is to help mothers make accurate risk-benefit comparisons by helping them balance the risks of being on medication and breastfeeding, the risk of not breastfeeding, and the risks to themselves and their babies of ongoing, untreated depression. Oftentimes, mothers make a false comparison of "contaminated" breast milk (i.e., by medications) with "pristine" formula. In almost all circumstances, the risks of breastfeeding while on medications are far less than the risk of not breastfeeding (Hale, 2010).

- Mothers may be more amenable to medications if they feel like there is an end-point. For example, some may be willing to take medications if there is a plan in place for evaluating them, say at 4 to 6 months, to see if they need to continue or can taper off. In the meantime, other treatments, such as exercise, therapy, or Omega-3s, can be put into place, so they are less vulnerable to future episodes.

B. Alternative Treatments

1. Long-Chain Omega-3 Fatty Acids: EPA and DHA

a.   EPA and DHA, the long-chain Omega-3 fatty acids, show promise in the treatment of mood disorders according to a 2006 expert panel convened by the American Psychiatric Association (Freeman et al., 2006a). DHA alone has some potential efficacy in preventing depression but not in treating it (Akabas & Deckelbaum, 2006; Kendall-Tackett, 2010c). EPA is effective for treatment of depression and can be used alone or in combination with either DHA or medications (Akabas & Deckelbaum, 2006; Peet & Stokes, 2005).

b.   Mothers from many industrialized countries are deficient in EPA and DHA because they do not consume enough in their diets. Pregnant and postpartum women are often especially deficient because the baby needs these fatty acids for its developing nervous system. Because of this, mothers' bodies will preferentially divert these fatty acids to the babies and the mothers become increasingly depleted with each subsequent pregnancy (Rees, Austin, & Parker, 2005).

c.   A population study from New Zealand found that the more fish people ate, the higher their self-reported mental health. This study controlled for other variables that could explain the results including age, household income, eating patterns, alcohol use, and smoking (Silvers & Scott, 2002).

d.   Hibbeln (2002) examined seafood consumption in more than 14,000 pregnant women. He found that women who ate high amounts of seafood while pregnant, and who had high levels of DHA in their milk postpartum, had lower levels of postpartum depression.

> ## Contaminant-Free Sources of EPA/DHA
>
> Brands of OTC Fish-Oil Supplements verified by the U.S. Pharmacopeia (checked for mercury, PCBs, and all major contaminants)
>
> www.USP.org
>
> ### Dosages
> - 200-400 mg of DHA is the current minimum recommended dose to prevent depression.
>
> - 1,000 mg EPA for treatment of depression usually in combination with medications and/or DHA.

e. Pregnant or breastfeeding women generally cannot safely consume enough seafood to achieve an antidepressant effect because contaminants in seafood are toxic to the baby's developing nervous system. Fortunately, there are supplements available that are tested for contaminants and are safe for pregnant and breastfeeding women (see Contaminant-Free Sources of EPA/DHA).

f. EPA/DHA decrease inflammation by lowering levels of proinflammatory cytokines. A large population study found that people with high levels of Omega-3s in their blood had low levels of proinflammatory cytokines. In contrast, people with low levels of Omega-3s had more pro-inflammatory cytokines (Ferrucci et al., 2006).

g. The Omega-3 in flax seed is ALA and does not have efficacy in the prevention or treatment of depression (Bratman & Girman, 2003).

2. Exercise

a. The effectiveness of exercise as a treatment for depression has been demonstrated in population studies and randomized clinical trials (Daley, Macarthur, & Winter, 2007).

b.   An Australian study of 587 new mothers (Su, Zhao, Binna, Scott, & Oddy, 2007) examined the relationship between mothers' exercise, initiation, and duration of breastfeeding, and exercise's effect on infant growth. Exercise had no negative effect on either breastfeeding or infant growth.

c.   In a Finnish population study (N=3,403), men and women who exercised two to three times a week experienced significantly less depression, anger, cynical distrust, and stress than men and women who exercised less frequently (Hassmen, Koivula, & Uutela, 2000).

d.   The efficacy of exercise as a treatment for major depressive disorder (MDD) was also demonstrated in two randomized trials. In the first study, 156 patients with MDD (>50 years old) were randomized into one of three treatment groups: aerobic exercise alone, sertraline (Zoloft) alone, and a combination of exercise and sertraline. After four months, both sertraline and exercise were effective in treating major depression with no significant difference between them (Babyak et al., 2000). This group of researchers replicated their findings with another group of depressed older patients. Exercise was as effective as sertraline for treating major depression (Blumenthal et al., 2007).

e.   In order to achieve an antidepressive effect, mothers with mild- to-moderate depression must exercise 2 to 3 times a week for 20 to 30 minutes at a moderate level. For major depression, 3 to 5 times a week is necessary for 45 to 60 minutes (Kendall-Tackett, 2008).

3. S-Adenosyl-L-Methionine (SAMe)

a.   S-Adenosyl-L-Methionine (SAMe) is another supplement that is effective in treating depression. SAMe is a substance that naturally occurs in every cell of the body and is crucial to cell metabolism in all animals. It is derived from the amino acid methionine and adenosine triphosphate.

b. SAMe contributes to a process known as methylation that regulates serotonin, melatonin, dopamine, and adrenaline. It also regulates neurotransmitter metabolism, membrane fluidity, and receptor activity (Bratman & Girman, 2003). If people have low levels of B6, B12, or folic acid, SAMe breaks down into homocysteine. High homocysteine levels are harmful to cardiovascular health and have been related to depression.

c. A meta-analysis of 28 studies indicated that SAMe decreased depression significantly more than a placebo, and was comparable to antidepressant medications in its effectiveness (Agency for Healthcare Research and Quality, 2002). The authors of this report noted that in placebo trials, SAMe was providing an active treatment. Clinically, patients improved, but SAMe did not completely eradicate depression.

d. Unfortunately, we have no information on the impact of SAMe on breastfeeding. Since it naturally occurs in the body, and has been safely used during pregnancy (Agency for Healthcare Research and Quality, 2002), it is most likely safe. However, we don't know that for certain and should advise mothers accordingly.

4. Other Alternative Treatments

a. At this point, there is not a large empirical base on the efficacy of other alternative treatments for postpartum depression. However, a recent review highlights some of the approaches that are promising, and should be considered as possible approaches to treating depressed mothers. Some of these other modalities include

Ayurvedic medicine, homeopathy, aromatherapy, massage, and Traditional Chinese Medicine (Mantle, 2002).

b. Bright light therapy was helpful in two case studies of new mothers (Corral, Kuan, & Kostaras, 2000). Both women refused to take antidepressants, but responded to bright light therapy and had significantly lower rates of depressive symptoms after treatment.

c. In a Finnish study of healthy adults (ages 26 to 63 years), patients were randomly assigned to one of three conditions: aerobics class with bright light, aerobics class with normal illumination, and relaxation/stretching sessions in bright light as a control group. The authors found that bright light and exercise relieved depression. For atypical depression, bright light was more effective than exercise. The authors concluded that twice-weekly administration of bright light, alone or with physical exercise, can alleviate seasonal depression (Leppaemaeki, Partonen, Hurme, Haukka, & Loennqvist, 2002).

A full set of handouts for mothers on exercise, Omega-3s, and bright light therapy is available at http://www.uppitysciencechick.com/ppdhandouts.html. These can be downloaded and shared for free.

C. Psychotherapy

- Two forms of therapy have proven efficacious for the treatment of mild, moderate or severe depression: cognitive-behavioral therapy and interpersonal psychotherapy.

- Both of these types of therapy have proven as effective as medications in randomized clinical trials, and have been used to treat postpartum women.

1. Cognitive-Behavioral Therapy

a. Cognitive-behavioral therapy (CBT) has been shown to be as effective as medications for treating depression, anxiety, chronic pain, obsessive compulsive disorder, and PTSD (International Society for Traumatic Stress Studies, 2009; Rupke, Blecke, & Renfrow, 2006).

b. CBT is based on the premise that depression is caused by distortions in thinking. The goal is to help patients learn to identify distorted beliefs and replace them with more rational ones (Rupke, 2006).

c. Patients who received CBT did better on follow-up, were less likely to relapse, and were less likely to drop out of treatment than those who received medications alone (Rupke et al., 2006). CBT has also proven effective for the treatment of depression in adolescents (Rupke et al., 2006).

d. Mothers may also try a self-help approach. *Feeling Good: The New Mood Therapy* by David Burns can help mothers who are interested in trying cognitive therapy, like to read, and don't have access to a therapist who offers cognitive-behavioral therapy. A simplified version, used in Dr. Burns' inner-city clinic, is *Ten Days to Self-Esteem*. (The title does not mention depression, but the purpose of this book was to provide the information in *Feeling Good* in a more accessible form.)

e. State or province psychological associations can provide names of therapists in their states who offer CBT, but these practitioners may or may not be aware of the needs of postpartum women. (See also the National Association for Cognitive-Behavioral Therapy, www.nacbt.org, for more information.)

2. Interpersonal Psychotherapy

a. Interpersonal Psychotherapy (IPT) is another type of psychotherapy that has demonstrated effectiveness in the treatment of depression (Klier, Muzik, Rosenblum, & Lenz, 2001). It will likely become the psychotherapy of choice for postpartum depression. In one study, IPT was as effective as tricyclic antidepressants and cognitive therapy, and was effective for almost 70% of the patients (Tolman, 2001). (See also www.interpersonalpsychotherapy.org)

b. IPT is based on attachment theory, is time-limited, and focuses on the client's interpersonal relationships. Disturbances in these relationships are hypothesized as being responsible for depression in general, as well as postpartum depression in particular (Stuart & O'Hara, 1995).

c. With IPT, on a client's first visit, a specific problem is identified, and the client and therapist begin working on that issue. The goal of IPT is to help new mothers combine their new roles with the ones they have already established. This might involve helping the mother solve a problem. But the actual solution is less important than the process of identifying a problem and making a change.

d. IPT was effective for postpartum depression in a study of 120 women with postpartum major depression (O'Hara et al., 2000). O'Hara et al. found that women in the therapy group had significantly lower depression scores than women in the waitlist group at 4, 8, and 12 weeks after completing treatment. IPT reduced depressive symptoms and improved social adjustment. The authors felt that IPT represents a viable alternative to pharmacotherapy, especially for women who are breastfeeding.

D. Medications

1. Herbal Medications

a.   St. John's wort *(Hypericum perforatum)* is an effective treatment for mild-to-moderate depression. It has also been effective for major depression, although, this is not its standard use.

b.   St. John's wort is the most widely used antidepressant in the world and has many other properties. It is antibacterial, anti-inflammatory, antiviral, and relieves pain (Balch, 2002; Ernst, 2002).

c.   A review of 22 studies (Whiskey, Werneke, & Taylor, 2001) found that St. John's wort was more effective than the placebo in treating depression, and did not significantly differ from standard antidepressants in its effectiveness. The authors also concluded that side effects were more common with standard antidepressants than with St. John's wort.

d.   In one study (Lecrubier, Clerc, Didi, & Kieser, 2002), 375 patients were randomized to receive either St. John's wort *(Hypericum perforatum* Extract WS 5570) or a placebo for mild-to-moderate depression. The patients received treatment for 6 weeks. At the end of 6 weeks, patients receiving St. John's wort had significantly lower scores on the Hamilton Depression Rating Scale, and significantly more patients were in remission or had a response to treatment, than patients receiving the placebo.

e.   St. John's wort was even effective with major depression. This study (Van Gurp, Meterissian, Haiek, McCusker, & Bellavance, 2002) included 87 patients with major depression recruited from Canadian family practice physicians. Patients were randomly assigned to receive either St. John's wort or sertraline. At the end of the 12-week trial, both groups improved, and there was no difference between the two groups. But there were significantly more side effects in the sertraline group at 2 and 4 weeks. The authors concluded that St. John's wort, because of its effectiveness and benign side effects, was a good first choice for a primary care population.

f.   A review of 38 controlled clinical trials and two meta-analyses on St. John's wort found its safety and side-effect profile to be better than standard antidepressants. The incidence of adverse events ranged from 0% to 6%—10 times lower than antidepressants (Schultz, 2006).

g.   St. John's wort is currently considered safe for breastfeeding mothers. But mothers should tell their doctors that they are taking it since it can interact with several classes of prescription medications including oral contraceptives, cyclosporins, and standard antidepressants (Hale, 2010; Schultz, 2006). It should never be combined with standard antidepressants.

h.   Kava, another herb that is sometimes paired with St. John's wort for treatment of anxiety, is sedative and interacts with several classes of medications, including benzodiazepines, alcohol, and antidepressants. There have been some case reports of liver damage and other toxic effects, but these are relatively rare (Hale, 2010).

i.   Kava is currently contraindicated for breastfeeding mothers (Balch, 2002; Hale, 2010).

2. Antidepressant Medications

a.   There are three major classes of antidepressants: tricyclics, selective serotonin reuptake inhibitors (SSRIs), and monoamine oxidase inhibitors (MAOIs). Only MAOIs are incompatible with breastfeeding.

b.   SSRIs are used most frequently in pregnant women and breastfeeding mothers (Beck, 2006; Hale, 2010).

c.   Medications with inert metabolites are preferred for breast-feeding mothers since they result in lower exposure of the baby to the medication. These include sertraline, escitalopram, and paroxetine. But there are some concerns about use of paroxetine during the first trimester of pregnancy, due to possible neonatal complications.

d.   For women taking SSRIs while breastfeeding, providers should watch infants for sedation, agitation, irritability, poor feeding, and gastrointestinal distress (Beck, 2006).

e.   Only one class of antidepressants—monoamine oxidase inhibitors (MAOIs)—is *always* contraindicated for breastfeeding mothers (e.g., Nardil, Parnate).

f.   For more current information about antidepressants and breastfeeding, go to the InfantRisk Center (www.infantrisk.org).

Appendix

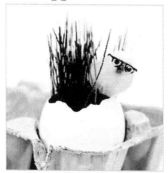

Postpartum Depression Predictors Inventory—Revised

Marital Status (Circle One)

- *Single*
- *Married/Cohabitating*
- *Separated*
- *Divorced*
- *Widowed*
- *Partnered*

Socioeconomic Status (Circle One)

- *Low*
- *Middle*
- *High*

During Pregnancy

Self-Esteem (Y/N)

- *Do you feel good about yourself as a person?*
- *Do you feel worthwhile?*
- *Do you feel you have a number of good qualities as a person?*

Prenatal Depression (Y/N)

Have you ever felt depressed during your pregnancy?

- *If yes, when and how long have you been feeling this way?*
- *If yes, how mild or severe would you consider your depression?*

Prenatal Anxiety (Y/N)

Have you ever felt anxious during your pregnancy?

- *If yes, how long have you been feeling this way?*

Unplanned/Unwanted Pregnancy (Y/N)

- *Was the pregnancy planned?*
- *Is the pregnancy unwanted?*

History of Previous Depression (Y/ N)

Before this pregnancy, have you ever been depressed?

- *If yes, when did you experience this depression?*
- *If yes, have you been under a physician's care for this depression?*
- *If yes, did the physician prescribe a medication for your depression?*

Marital Satisfaction (Y/N)

- *Are you satisfied with your marriage (or living arrangement)?*
- *Are you currently experiencing any marital problems?*
- *Are things going well between you and your partner?*

Social Support (Y/N)

- *Do you feel you receive adequate support from your partner?*
- *Do you feel you receive adequate instrumental support from your partner? (such as help with household chores or babysitting)*
- *Do you feel you can rely on your partner when you need help?*
- *Do you feel you can confide in your partner?*

Repeat questions for family and friends.

Life Stress (Y/N)

Are you currently experiencing any stressful events in your life such as:

- *Financial problems? Marital problems? Death in the family? Serious illness in the family? Moving? Unemployment? Job change?*

After Delivery, Add the Following Items

Child Care Stress (Y/N)

- *Is your infant experiencing any health problems?*
- *Are you having problems with your baby feeding?*
- *Are you having problems with your baby sleeping?*

Infant Temperament (Y/N)

- *Would you consider your baby irritable or fussy?*
- *Does your baby cry a lot?*
- *Is your baby difficult to console or soothe?*

Maternity Blues (Y/N)

- *Did you experience a brief period of tearfulness and mood swings during the first week after delivery?*

Reprinted with permission from Beck, C.T. (2006). Postpartum depression: It isn't just the blues. *American Journal of Nursing, 106*, 40-50.

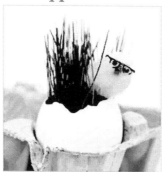

Edinburgh Postnatal Depression Scale (EPDS)

The Edinburgh Postnatal Depression Scale (EPDS) has been developed to assist primary care health professionals to detect mothers suffering from postnatal depression; a distressing disorder more prolonged than the "blues" (which occur in the first week after delivery), but less severe than puerperal psychosis.

Previous studies have shown that postnatal depression affects at least 10% of women and that many depressed mothers remain untreated. These mothers may cope with their baby and with household tasks, but their enjoyment of life is seriously affected and it is possible that there are long-term effects on the family.

The EPDS was developed at health centers in Livingston and Edinburgh. It consists of 10 short statements. The mother underlines which of the four possible responses is closest to how she has been feeling during the past week. Most mothers complete the scale without difficulty in less than five minutes.

The validation study showed that mothers who scored above a threshold of 12/13 were likely to be suffering from a depressive illness of varying severity. Nevertheless, the EPDS score should not override clinical judgment. A careful clinical as sessment should be carried out to confirm the diagnosis. The scale indicates how the mother has felt during the previous week, and in doubtful cases, it may be usefully repeated after two weeks. The scale will not detect mothers with anxiety neuroses, phobias, or personality disorders.

Instructions for Users

1. The mother is asked to underline the response which comes closest to how she has been feeling in the previous 7 days.

2. All 10 items must be completed.

3. Care should be taken to avoid the possibility of the mother discussing her answers with others.

4. The mother should complete the scale herself, unless she has limited English or has difficulty with reading.

5. The EPDS may be used at 6-8 weeks to screen postnatal women. The child health clinic, postnatal check-up, or a home visit may provide suitable opportunities for its completion.

Scoring

Response categories are scored 0, 1, 2, and 3 according to increased severity of the symptom. Items marked with an asterisk are reverse scored (i.e., 3, 2, 1, and 0). The total score is calculated by adding together the scores for each of the 10 items.

Reprinted with permission from: Cox, J.L., Holder, J.M., & Sagovsky, R. (1987). Detection of postnatal depression: Development of the 10-item Edinburgh Postnatal Depression Scale. *British Journal of Psychiatry, 150, 782-786.*

EPDS

As you have recently had a baby, we would like to know how you are feeling. Please UNDERLINE the answer which comes closest to how you have felt IN THE PAST 7 DAYS, not just how you feel today. Here is an example already completed.

I have felt happy...

- *Yes, all the time*
- *<u>Yes, most of the time</u>*
- *No, not very often*
- *No, not at all*

In the past 7 days...

1. **I have been able to laugh and see the funny side of things:**
   - *As much as I always have*
   - *Not quite so much now*
   - *Definitely not so much now*
   - *Not at all*

2. **I have looked forward with enjoyment to things:**
   - *As much as I ever did*
   - *Somewhat less than I used to*
   - *Definitely less than I used to*
   - *Hardly at all*

* 3. **I have blamed myself unnecessarily when things went wrong:**
   - *Yes, most of the time*
   - *Yes, some of the time*
   - *Not very often*
   - *No, never*

4. **I have been anxious or worried for no good reason:**
   - *No, not at all*
   - *Hardly ever*
   - *Yes, sometimes*
   - *Yes, very often*

* 5. **I have felt scared or panicky for no very good reason:**
   - *Yes, quite a lot*
   - *Yes, sometimes*
   - *No, not much*
   - *No, not at all*

* 6. **Things have been getting on top of me:**
   - *Yes, most of the time, I haven't been able to cope at all*
   - *Yes, sometimes, I haven't been coping as well as usual*
   - *No, I have been coping as well as ever*
   - *No, most of the time I have coped quite well*

* 7. **I have been so unhappy that I have had difficulty sleeping:**
   - *Yes, most of the time*
   - *Yes, sometimes*
   - *Not very often*
   - *No, not at all*

* 8. **I have felt sad or miserable:**
   - *Yes, most of the time*
   - *Yes, quite often*
   - *Not very often*
   - *No, not at all*

* 9. **I have been so unhappy that I have been crying:**
  - *Yes, most of the time*
  - *Yes, quite often*
  - *Only occasionally*
  - *No, never*

* 10. **The thought of harming myself has occurred to me:**
  - *Yes, quite often*
  - *Sometimes*
  - *Hardly ever*
  - *Never*

Appendix C

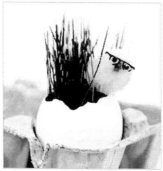

Other Depression Resources

- **Praeclarus Press** (www.PraeclarusPress.com)

- **Uppity Science Chick** (www.uppitysciencechick.com)

- **NH Breastfeeding Task Force** (www.NHBreastfeedingTaskForce.org)

- **Breastfeeding Made Simple** (www.BreastfeedingMadeSimple.com)

- **Academy of Breastfeeding Medicine** (www.bfmed.org)

- **Postpartum Support International** (www.postpartum.net)

References

Abramowitz, J. S., Schwartz, S. A., Moore, K., Carmin, C., Wiegartz, P. S., & Purdon, C. (2002). Obsessive-compulsive symptoms in pregnancy and the puerperium: A review of the literature. *Anxiety Disorders, 87,* 49-74.

Agency for Healthcare Research and Quality. (2002). *S-Adenosyl-L-Methionine for treatment of depression, osteoarthritis, and live disease.* Rockville, MD: U.S. Department of Health and Human Services.

Ahokas, A., Aito, M., & Rimon, R. (2000). Positive treatment effect of estradiol in postpartum psychosis: A pilot study. *Journal of Clinical Psychiatry, 61,* 166-169.

Ahokas, A., Kaukoranta, J., Wahlbeck, K., & Aito, M. (2001). Estrogen deficiency in severe postpartum depression: Successful treatment with sublingual physiologic 17-beta estradiol: A preliminary study. *Journal of Clinical Psychiatry, 62,* 332-336.

Akabas, S. R., & Deckelbaum, R. J. (2006). Summary of a workshop on n-3 fatty acids: Current status of recommendations and future directions. *American Journal of Clinical Nutrition, 83,* 1536-1538.

Alcorn, K. L., O'Donovan, A., Patrick, J. C., Creedy, D., & Devilly, G. J. (2010). A prospective longitudinal study of the prevalence of post-traumatic stress disorder resulting from childbirth events. *Psychological Medicine, 40,* 1849-1859.

Amir, L. H., Dennerstein, L., Garland, S. M., Fisher, J., & Farish, S. J. (1996). Psychological aspects of nipple pain in lactating women. *Journal of Psychosomatic Obstetrics & Gynecology, 17,* 53-58.

Babyak, M., Blumenthal, J. A., Herman, S., Khatri, P., Doraiswamy, M., Moore, K.,…Krishnan, R. R. (2000). Exercise treatment for major depression: Maintenance of therapeutic benefit at 10 months. *Psychosomatic Medicine, 62,* 633-638.

Balch, P. (2002). *Prescription for herbal healing.* New York: Avery.

Beck, C. T. (2001). Predictors of postpartum depression: An update. *Nursing Research, 50,* 275-285.

Beck, C. T. (2004a). Birth trauma: In the eye of the beholder. *Nursing Research, 53*(1), 28-35.

Beck, C. T. (2004b). Posttraumatic stress disorder due to childbirth. *Nursing Research, 53,* 216-224.

Beck, C. T. (2006). Postpartum depression: It isn't just the blues. *American Journal of Nursing, 106*(5), 40-50.

Beck, C. T., & Gable, R. K. (2000). Postpartum Depression Screening Scale: Development and psychometric testing. *Nursing Research, 49,* 272-282.

Beck, C. T., Gable, R. K., Sakala, C., & Declercq, E. R. (2011). Posttraumatic stress disorder in new mothers: Results from a two-stage U.S. national survey. *Birth, 38*(3), 216-227.

Beck, C. T., & Watson, S. (2008). Impact of birth trauma on breastfeeding. *Nursing Research, 57*(4), 228-236.

Benedict, M. I., Paine, L., & Paine, L. (1994). *Long-term effects of child sexual abuse on functioning in pregnancy and pregnancy outcomes (Final Report).* Washington, DC: National Center of Child Abuse & Neglect.

Blumenthal, J. A., Babyak, M. A., Doraiswamy, P. M., Watkins, L., Hoffman, B. M., & Barbour, K. A., et al. (2007). Exercise and pharmacotherapy in the treatment of major depressive disorder. *Psychosomatic Medicine, 69,* 587-596.

Bratman, S., & Girman, A. M. (2003). *Handbook of herbs and supplements and their therapeutic uses.* St Louis: Mosby.

Brennan, P. A., Hammen, C., Anderson, M.J., Bor, W., Najman, J.M., & Williams, G.M. (2000). Chronicity, severity, and timing of maternal depressive symptoms: Relationships with child outcomes at age 5. *Developmental Psychology, 36,* 759-766.

Buss, C., Davis, E. P., Shahbaba, B., Pruessner, J. C., Head, K., & Sandman, C. A. (2012). Maternal cortisol over the course of pregnancy and subsequent child amygdala and hippocampus volumes and affecive problems. *Proceedings of the National Academy of Sciences USA, 109*(20), E1312-E1319.

Centers for Disease Control. (2008). Prevalence of postpartum depressive symptoms: 17 states, 2004-2005. *Morbidity & Mortality Weekly Report, 57*(14), 361-367.

Corral, M., Kuan, A., & Kostaras, D. (2000). Bright light therapy's effect on postpartum depression. *American Journal of Psychiatry, 157,* 303-304.

Corwin, E. J., Bozoky, I., Pugh, L. C., & Johnston, N. (2003). Interleukin-1 beta elevation during the postpartum period. *Annals of Behavioral Medicine, 25,* 41-47.

Corwin, E. J., & Pajer, K. (2008). The psychoneuroimmunology of postpartum depression. *Journal of Women's Health, 17*(9), 1529-1534.

Coussons-Read, M. E., Okun, M. L., Schmitt, M. P., & Giese, S. (2005). Prenatal stress alters cytokine levels in a manner that may endanger human pregnancy. *Psychosomatic Medicine, 67,* 625-631.

Cox, J. L., Holden, J. M., & Sagovsky, R. (1987). Detection of postnatal depression: Development of the 10-item Edinburgh Postnatal Depression Scale. *British Journal of Psychiatry, 150,* 782-786.

Daley, A. J., Macarthur, C., & Winter, H. (2007). The role of exercise in treating postpartum depression: A review of the literature. *Journal of Midwifery and Women's Health, 52,* 56-62.

Dayan, J., Creveuil, C., Marks, M.N., Conroy, S., Herlicoviez, M., Dreyfus, M., & Tordjman, S. (2006). Prenatal depression, prenatal anxiety, and spontaneous preterm birth: A prospective cohort study among women with early and regular care. *Psychosomatic Medicine, 68,* 938-946.

Declercq, E. R., Sakala, C., Corry, M. P., & Applebaum, S. (2008). *New mothers speak out: National survey results highlight women's postpartum experiences.* New York: Childbirth Connection.

Dennis, C.-L., & McQueen, K. (2009). The relationship between infant-feeding outcomes and postpartum depression: A qualitative systematic review. *Pediatrics, 123,* e736-e751.

Eisenach, J. c., Pan, P. H., Smiley, R., Lavand'homme, P., Landau, R., & Houle, T. T. (2008). Severity of acute pain after childbirth, but not type of delivery, predicts persistent pain and postpartum depression. *Pain, 140,* 87-94.

Elmir, R., Schmied, V., Wilkes, L., & Jackson, D. (2010). Women's perceptions and experiences of a traumatic birth: A meta-ethnography. *Journal of Advanced Nursing, 66*(10), 2142-2153.

Ernst, E. (2002). The risk-benefit profile of commonly used herbal therapies: Ginkgo, St. John's wort, ginseng, echinacea, saw palmetto, and kava. *Annals of Internal Medicine, 136,* 42-53.

Evans, J., Heron, J., Francomb, H., Oke, S., & Golding, J. (2001). Cohort study of depressed mood during pregnancy and after childbirth. *British Medical Journal, 323,* 257-260.

Feeley, N., Zelkowitz, P., Cormier, C., Charbonneau, L., Lacroix, A., & Papgeorgiou, A. (2011). Posttraumatic stress among mother of very low birthweight infants 6 months after discharge from the neonatal intensive care unit. *Applied Nursing Research, 24,* 114-117.

Feldman, R., Eidelman, A. I., Sirota, L., & Weller, A. (2002). Comparison of skin-to-skin (kangaroo) and traditional care: parenting outcomes and preterm infant development. *Pediatrics, 110*(1 Pt 1), 16-26.

Fergusson, D. M., Boden, J. M., & Horwood, L. J. (2008). Exposure to childhood sexual and physical abuse and adjustment in early adulthood. *Child Abuse & Neglect, 32,* 607-619.

Ferrucci, L., Cherubini, A., Bandinelli, S., Bartali, B., Corsi, A., Lauretani, F.,...Guralnik, J. M. (2006). Relationship of plasma polyunsaturated fatty acids to circulating inflammatory markers. *Journal of Clinical Endocrinology & Metabolism, 91,* 439-446.

Field, T., Diego, M., Hernandez-Reif, M., Figueiredo, B., Schanberg, S., & Kuhn, C. (2007). Sleep disturbance in depressed pregnant women and their newborns. *Infant Behavior & Development, 30,* 127-133.

Franko, D. L., Blais, M. A., Becker, A. E., Delinsky, S. S., Greenwood, D. N., Flores, A. T.,...Herzog, D. B. (2001). Pregnancy complications and neonatal outcomes in women with eating disorders. *American Journal of Psychiatry, 158,* 1461-1466.

Freeman, M. P., Hibbeln, J. R., Wisner, K. L., Davis, J. M., Mischoulon, D., Peet, M.,...Stoll, A. L. (2006a). Omega-3 fatty acids: Evidence basis for treatment and future research in psychiatry. *Journal of Clinical Psychiatry, 67,* 1954-1967.

Friedman, M. J., Resick, P. A., Bryant, R. A., & Brewin, C. R. (2011). Considering PTSD for DSM-5. *Depression & Anxiety, 28,* 750-769.

Galea, S., Vlahov, D., Resnick, H., Ahern, J., Susser, E., Gold, J.,... Kilpatrick, D. (2003). Trends of probable post-traumatic stress disorder in New York City after the September 11 terrorist attacks. *American Journal of Epidemiology, 158,* 514-524.

Gaynes, B. N., Gavin, N., Meltzer-Brody, S., Lohr, K. N., Swinson, T., Gartlehner, G.,...Miller, W. C. (2005). *Perinatal depression: Prevalence, screening, accuracy, and screening outcomes.* Agency for Healthcare Research and Quality, AHRQ Pub. No. 05-E006-1(119).

Gjerdingen, D., Crow, S., McGovern, P., Miner, M., & Center, B. (2009). Postpartum depression screening at well-child visits: Validity of a 2-question screen and the PHQ-9. *Annals of Family Medicine, 7*(1), 63-70.

Goyal, D., Gay, C. L., & Lee, K. A. (2007). Patterns of sleep disruption and depressive symptoms in new mothers. *Journal of Perinatal & Neonatal Nursing, 21*(2), 123-129.

Grajeda, R., & Perez-Escamilla, R. (2002). Stress during labor and delivery is associated with delayed onset of lactation among urban Guatemalan women. *Journal of Nutrition, 132,* 3055-3060.

Grant, K.-A., McMahon, C., Austin, M.-P., Reilly, N., Leader, L., & Ali, S. (2009). Maternal prenatal anxiety, postnatal caregiving and infants' cortisol responss to the still-face procedure. *Developmental Psychobiology, 51,* 625-637.

Groër, M., Davis, K., & Casey, B. (2005). Neuroendocrine and immune relationships in postpartum fatigue. *MCN, 30*, 133-138.

Groër, M. W., Davis, M. W., Smith, K. W., Casey, K., Kramer, V., & Bukovsky, E. (2005). Immunity, inflammation and infection in post-partum breast and formula feeders. *American Journal of Reproductive Immunology, 54*, 222-231.

Hale, T. W. (2010). *Medications and mothers' milk, 14th Edition.* Amarillo, TX: Hale Publishing.

Hammen, C., & Brennan, P. (2002). Interpersonal dysfunction in depressed women: Impairments independent of depressive symptoms. *Journal of Affective Disorders, 72*, 145-156.

Hassmen, P., Koivula, N., & Uutela, A. (2000). Physical exercise and psychological well-being: A population study in Finland. *Preventative Medicine, 30*, 17-25.

Heneghan, A. M., Chaudron, L. H., Storfer-Isser, A., Park, E. R., Kelleher, K. J., Stein, R. E. K. (2007). Factors associated with identification and management or maternal depression by pediatricians. *Pediatrics, 119*, 44-454.

Hibbeln, J. R. (2002). Seafood consumption, the DHA content of mothers' milk and prevalence rates of postpartum depression: A cross-national, ecological analysis. *Journal of Affective Disorders, 69*, 15-29.

International Society for Traumatic Stress Studies (Ed.). (2009). *Effective treatments for PTSD: Psychopharmacology for adults (Guideline 6).* New York: Guilford.

Jones, N. A., McFall, B. A., & Diego, M. A. (2004). Patterns of brain electrical activity in infants of depressed mothers who breastfeed and bottle feed: The mediating role of infant temperament. *Biological Psychology, 67*, 103-124.

Jotzo, M., & Poets, C. F. (2005). Helping parents cope with the trauma of premature birth: An evaluation of a trauma-preventive psychological intervention. *Pediatrics, 115*, 915-919.

Kabir, K., Sheeder, J., & Kelly, L. S. (2008). Identifying postpartum depression: Are 3 questions as good as 10? *Pediatrics, 122,* e696-e702.

Kendall-Tackett, K. A. (2007). A new paradigm for depression in new mothers: The central role of inflammation and how breastfeeding and anti-inflammatory treatments protect maternal mental health. *International Breastfeeding Journal, 2:6.* doi: doi:10.1186/1746-4358-2-6

Kendall-Tackett, K. A. (2008). *Non-pharmacologic treatments for depression in new mothers.* Amarillo, TX: Hale Publishing.

Kendall-Tackett, K. A. (2010a). Breastfeeding beats the blues. *Mothering, Sept/Oct,* 60-69.

Kendall-Tackett, K. A. (2010b). *Depression in new mothers: Causes, consequences and treatment options, 2nd Edition.* London: Routledge.

Kendall-Tackett, K. A. (2010c). Long-chain omega-3 fatty acids and women's mental health in the perinatal period. *Journal of Midwifery and Women's Health, 55*(6), 561-567.

Kendall-Tackett, K. A. (2013). *Treating the lifetime health effects of childhood victimization, 2nd Edition.* Kingston, NJ: Civic Research Institute.

Kendall-Tackett, K. A. (2014a). Childbirth-related posttraumatic stress disorder symptoms and implications for breastfeeding. *Clinical Lactation, 5*(2), 51-55.

Kendall-Tackett, K. A. (2014b). Intervention for mothers who have experienced childbirth-related trauma and posttraumatic stress disorder. *Clinical Lactation, 5*(2), 56-61.

Kendall-Tackett, K. A., Cong, Z., & Hale, T. W. (2011). The effect of feeding method on sleep duration, maternal well-being, and postpartum depression. *Clinical Lactation, 2*(2), 22-26.

Kendall-Tackett, K. A., Cong, Z., & Hale, T. W. (2013). Depression, sleep quality, and maternal well-being in postpartum women with a history of sexual assault: A comparison of breastfeeding, mixed-feeding, and formula-feeding mothers. *Breastfeeding Medicine, 8*(1), 16-22.

Kiecolt-Glaser, J. K., Belury, M. A., Porter, K., Beversdoft, D., Lemeshow, S., & Glaser, R. (2007). Depressive symptoms, omega-6: omega-3 fatty acids, and inflammation in older adults. *Psychosomatic Medicine, 69,* 217-224.

Klier, C. M., Muzik, M., Rosenblum, K. L., & Lenz, G. (2001). Interpersonal psychotherapy adapted for the group setting in the treatment of postpartum depression. *Journal of Psychotherapy Practice and Research, 10,* 124-131.

Knipscheer, J. W., & Kleber, R. J. (2006). The relative contribution of posttraumatic and acculturative stress to subjective mental health among Bosnian refugees. *Journal of Clinical Psychology, 62(3),* 339-353.

Konsman, J. P., Parnet, P., & Dantzer, R. (2002). Cytokine-induced sickness behaviour: Mechanisms and implications. *Trends in Neuroscience, 25,* 154-158.

Kop, W. J., & Gottdiener, J. S. (2005). The role of immune system parameters in the relationship between depression and coronary artery disease. *Psychosomatic Medicine, 67,* S37-S41.

Lecrubier, Y., Clerc, G., Didi, R., & Kieser, M. (2002). Efficacy of St. John's wort extract WS 5570 in major depression: A double-blind, placebo-controlled trial. *American Journal of Psychiatry, 159,* 1361-1366.

Lee, S.-Y., Lee, K. A., Rankin, S. H., Weiss, S. J., & Alkon, A. (2007). Sleep disturbance, fatigue, and stress among Chinese-American parents with ICU hospitalized infants. *Issues in Mental Health Nursing, 28,* 593-605.

Leppaemaeki, S. J., Partonen, T. T., Hurme, J., Haukka, J. K., & Loennqvist, J. K. (2002). Randomized trial of the efficacy of bright-light exposure and aerobic exercise on depressive symptoms and serum lipids. *Journal of Clinical Psychiatry, 63,* 316-321.

Lesperance, F., & Frasure-Smith, N. (2000). Depression in patients with cardiac disease: A practical review. *Journal of Psychosomatic Research, 48,* 379-391.

Luoma, I., Tamminen, T., Kaukonen, P., Laippala, P., Puura, K., Salelin, R., & Almqvist, F. (2001). Longitudinal study of maternal depressive symptoms and child well-being. *Journal of the American Academy of Child and Adolescent Psychiatry, 40*, 1367-1374.

Maes, M., & Smith, R.S. (1998). Fatty acids, cytokines, and major depression. *Biological Psychiatry, 43*, 313-314.

Maes, M., Bosmans, E., & Ombelet, W. (2004). In the puerperium, primiparae exhibit higher levels of anxiety and serum peptidase activity and greater immune responses than multiparae. *Journal of Clincal Psychiatry, 65*(1), 71-76.

Mantle, F. (2002). The role of alternative medicine in treating postnatal depression. *Complementary Therapies in Nursing and Midwifery, 8*, 197-203.

McKee, M. D., Cunningham, M., Jankowski, K. R., & Zayas, L. (2001). Health-related functional status in pregnancy: Relationship to depression and social support in a multi-ethnic population. *Obstetrics & Gynecology, 97*, 988-993.

Modarres, M., Afrasiabi, S., Rahnama, P., & Montazeri, A. (2012). Prevalence and risk factors of childbirth-related post-traumatic stress symptoms. *BMC Pregnancy and Childbirth, 12*(88). doi: http://www.biomedcentral.com/1471-2393/12/88

Oddy, W. H., Kendall, G. E., Li, J., Jacoby, P., Robinson, M., de Klerk, N. H.,...Stanley, F. J. (2009). The long-term effects of breastfeeding on child and adolescent mental health: A pregnancy cohort study followed for 14 years. *Journal of Pediatrics, 156*(4), 568-574.

Olfson, M., Marcus, S. C., Tedeschi, M., & Wan, G. J. (2006). Continuity of antidepressant treatment for adults with depression in the United States. American Journal of Psychiatry, 163, 101-108.

Orr, S. T., Reiter, J.P., Blazer, D.G., & James, S.A. (2007). Maternal prenatal pregnancy-related anxiety and spontaneous preterm birth in Baltimore, Maryland. *Psychosomatic Medicine, 69*, 566-570.

Peet, M., & Stokes, C. (2005). Omega-3 fatty acids in the treatment of psychiatric disorders. *Drugs, 65*, 1051-1059.

Posmontier, B. (2008). Sleep quality in women with and without postpartum depression. *Journal of Obstetric, Gynecologic and Neonatal Nursing, 37*(6), 722-737.

Prentice, J. C., Lu, M. C., Lange, L., & Halfon, N. (2002). The association between reported childhood sexual abuse and breastfeeding initiation. *Journal of Human Lactation, 18,* 291-226.

Rees, A.-M., Austin, M.-P., & Parker, G. (2005). Role of omega-3 fatty acids as a treatment for depression in the perinatal period. *Australia & New Zealand Journal of Psychiatry, 39,* 274-280.

Robles, T. F., Glaser, R., & Kiecolt-Glaser, J. K. (2005). Out of balance: A new look at chronic stress, depression, and immunity. *Current Directions in Psychological Science, 14,* 111-115.

Roux, G., Anderson, C., & Roan, C. (2002). Postpartum depression, marital dysfunction, and infant outcome: A longitudinal study. *Journal of Perinatal Education, 11,* 25-36.

Rowlands, I. J., & Redshaw, M. (2012). Mode of birth and women's psychological and physical wellbeing in the postnatal period. *BMC Pregnancy and Childbirth, 12*(138). doi: http://www.biomedcentral. com/1471-2393/12/138

Ruglass, L., & Kendall-Tackett, K. A. (2015). *The Psychology of Trauma 101.* New York: Springer.

Rupke, S. J., Blecke, D., & Renfrow, M. (2006). Cognitive therapy for depression. *American Family Physician, 73,* 83-86.

Schultz, V. (2006). Safety of St. John's wort extract compared to synthetic antidepressants. *Phytomedicine, 13,* 199-204.

Seng, J. S., Kohn-Wood, L. P., McPherson, M. D., & Sperlich, M. A. (2011). Disparity in posttraumatic stress disorder diagnosis among African American pregnant women. *Archives of Women's Mental Health, 14*(4), 295-306.

Seng, J. S., Low, L. K., Sperlich, M. A., Ronis, D. L., & Liberzon, I. (2011). Posttraumatic stress disorder, child abuse history, birth weight, and gestational age: A prospective cohort study. *British*

Journal of Obstetrics & Gynecology, 118(11), 1329-1339.

Silvers, K. M., & Scott, K. M. (2002). Fish consumption and self-reported physical and mental health status. *Public Health Nutrition, 5,* 427-431.

Soderquist, I., Wijma, B., Thorbert, G., & Wijma, K. (2009). Risk factors in pregnancy for post-traumatic stress and depression after childbirth. *British Journal of Obstetrics & Gynecology, 116,* 672-680.

Stern, G., & Kruckman, L. (1983). Multi-disciplinary perspectives on postpartum depression: An anthropological critique. *Social Science & Medicine, 17,* 1027-1041.

Stramrood, C. A., Paarlberg, K. M., Huis Veld, E. M., Berger, L. W. A. R., Vingerhoets, A. J. J. M., Schultz, W. C. M. W., & Van Pampus, M. G. (2011). Posttraumatic stress following childbirth in home-like- and hospital settings. *Journal of Psychosomatic Obstetrics & Gynecology, 32*(2), 88-97.

Strathearn, L., Mamun, A. A., Najman, J. M., & O'Callaghan, M. J. (2009). Does breastfeeding protect against substantiated child abuse and neglect? A 15-year cohort study. *Pediatrics, 123*(2), 483-493. doi: 123/2/483 [pii] 10.1542/peds.2007-3546

Stuart, S., & O'Hara, M. W. (1995). Interpersonal psychotherapy for postpartum depression. *Journal of Psychotherapy Practice and Research, 4,* 18-29.

Su, D., Zhao, Y., Binna, C., Scott, J., & Oddy, W. (2007). Breast-feeding mothers can exercise: Results of a cohort study. *Public Health Nutrition, 10,* 1089-1093.

Tolman, A. O. (2001). *Depression in adults: The latest assessment and treatment strategies.* Kansas City, MO: Compact Clinicals.

U.S. Department of Health and Human Services. (2011). *The Surgeon General's Call to Action to Support Breastfeeding.* Washington, DC: Author.

Van Gurp, G., Meterissian, G. B., Haiek, L. N., McCusker, J., & Bellavance, F. (2002). St. John's wort or sertraline?: Randomized controlled trial in primary care. *Canadian Family Physician, 48,* 905-912.

Walker, E. R., McGee, R. E., & Druss, B. G. (2015). Mortality in mental disorders and Global Disease Burden Implications: A systematic review and meta-analysis. *JAMA Psychiatry.* doi: 10.1001/jamapsychiatry.2014.2502

Watkins, S., Meltzer-Brody, S., Zolnoun, D., & Stuebe, A. M. (2011). Early breastfeeding experiences and postpartum depression *Obstetrics & Gynecology, 118*(2), 214-221.

Weissman, M. M., Wickramaratne, P., Nomura, Y., Warner, V., Pilowsky, D., & Verdeli, H. (2006). Offspring of depressed parents: 20 years later. *American Journal of Psychiatry, 163,* 1001-1008.

Whiskey, E., Werneke, U., & Taylor, D. (2001). A systematic review and meta-analysis of *Hypericum perforatum* in depression: A comprehensive clinical review. *International Clinical Psychopharmacology, 16,* 239-252.